HORMONES,
HOT FLASHES
AND
MOOD SWINGS

HORMONES, HOT FLASHES AND MOOD SWINGS

THE *MENOPAUSE* SURVIVAL GUIDE

CLARK GILLESPIE, M.D.

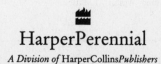

HarperPerennial
A Division of HarperCollinsPublishers

Grateful acknowledgment is made to John Johnson Ltd. for permission to reprint "Warning," © Jenny Joseph, from *Rose in the Afternoon,* Dent, 1974.

Originally published in 1989 by Harper & Row, Publishers, Inc.

HarperCollins books may be purchased for educational, business, or sales promotional use. For information please write: Special Markets Department, HarperCollins Publishers, Inc., 10 East 53rd Street, New York, NY 10022.

FIRST EDITION

Designed by Alma Orenstein

Library of Congress Cataloging-in-Publication Data

Gillespie, Clark.
    Hormones, hot flashes and mood swings : the menopause survival guide / Clark Gillespie.—Rev. ed.
       p. cm.
    Previously published: New York : Perennial Library, 1989.
    Includes index.
    ISBN 0-06-095017-X
    1. Menopause—Popular works. I. Title.
RG186.G54 1994
618.1′75—dc20   93-39092

98 97 96   RRD(H) 10 9 8 7 6 5 4

FOR MY BELOVED WIFE, *Susan*

When I am an old woman I shall wear purple
With a red hat which doesn't go, and doesn't suit me.
And I shall spend my pension on brandy and summer gloves
And satin sandals and say we've no money for butter.
I shall sit down on the pavement when I'm tired
And gobble up samples in shops and press alarm bells
And run my stick along the public railings
And make up for the sobriety of my youth.
I shall go out in my slippers in the rain
And pick the flowers in other people's gardens
And learn to spit . . .
But maybe I ought to practise a little now?
So people who know me are not too shocked and surprised
When suddenly I am old, and start to wear purple.

—JENNY JOSEPH

CONTENTS

PREFACE TO THE REVISED EDITION

The original introduction to our book—written in 1988—still stands intact and the four basic points it is built around remain unchallenged. Of course, there is a greatly expanded legion of menopausal and postmenopausal women now, and a great deal more research is being conducted on their behalf. In regard to that research, the North American Menopause Society—of which I am proud to be a founding member—has just entered a vast study of menopausal hormone replacement in conjunction with the NIH. But there are a great number of other promising things going on as we shall see in the next few years.

This preface to the new edition is written to summarize most of the important information that I have added to further your understanding of these important years. Our book has become more of a guide to all of your future health and safety concerns rather than just another menopause book. That is surely my goal.

Here's what's new:

- Your nutritional goals have been modified in light of the new food pyramid.

- The fitness information now stresses more active exercise and more resistance training.

- A completely new section, Gentlemen's Quarters, was written to help the man in your life understand the profound nature of your menopause.

- A much deeper look at breast disease and the new Tamoxifen study along with a new section on the diagnosis and management of ovarian cancer has been added.

- An update on osteoporosis and a totally new section on arteriosclerosis, a major postmenopausal threat, have been included.

- The new edition incorporates more information on the aging process and how to control it.

- Finally, hormone replacement therapy—including the use of testosterone—is brought into new focus.

Our human *life span* remains unchanged at eighty-five years. Some of us surpass that age, most do not. Nothing on the horizon is likely to push that limit farther away. Human *life expectancy,* however, is increasing in America. Thus, women reading this book who are in reasonable health can expect to live to their eighties.

Our goal is to live all these years in reasonable health and freedom—freedom to live where we wish, to move about, make our own decisions, and to enjoy what we do. That depends a great deal upon our lifestyle.

Our book—your book—helps you design a lifestyle that will push degenerative, restrictive problems into your future and compress them as much as you possibly can, to the close of life's journey.

The keys to our kingdom include:

- Fitness

- Nutrition

- Hormone Replacement Therapy

- Habit Control

- The Power to Do These Things

Let's go to health together!

INTRODUCTION

Four facts relating to women and aging have now become abundantly and unequivocally clear. First, life expectancy for women has increased dramatically in the United States during this century. Second, women are not only living longer, but are living healthier lives. This is due in part to improved lifestyles and in part to quality lifetime medical care, which has mitigated many of the potentially lethal and crippling disorders that at one time commonly afflicted women. Third, a fresh, reasonably healthy four million recruits are added each year to the more than forty million women presently living in the menopausal continuum. And one woman in seven will be over sixty-five by the turn of the century. All menopausal women will, of course, pass on. But that moment is being pushed farther away all the time, and as a result the menopausal and postmenopausal society continues to grow. Finally, and most important, menopause and the years that follow have been clearly established as an endocrine deficiency state—a disorder worthy of, and indeed, almost always requiring, comprehensive treatment.

Based on the preceding facts, this handbook has been written for, and is addressed to, all those women struggling through the menopause years. It is to serve as a companion and guide while you experience this tremendous journey—which, like all explorations, has its peaks and valleys, dangers and delights, dead ends and vistas, and which, without compass points, can lead to arid sand and stone rather than milk, honey and wine. Very clearly, these years can be savored or suffered, depending upon the route with which you are provided and whether or not you choose to follow it. The menopausal journey is a continuous one—always slightly uphill or downhill, but with some neat plateaus. In these pages I try to provide a gentle and compassionate compass for your journey.

HORMONES, HOT FLASHES *AND* MOOD SWINGS

1

THE FRUITFUL YEARS

The human menstrual life can be compared, with safety, to the life of a rose. Both lie dormant as the host grows, begin to bud in the exuberance of youth, flower in the fullness of adulthood, bear fruit for a generation and then draw back to support newer buds along the stem. And although a rose is supposedly sweeter in the bud than in full bloom, nothing is more exquisite than the fragrance of an open rose—particularly an open autumn rose—and, to prolong the floral allegory further, long after the bloom is off the rose, the attar of its petals lives on to perfume the days of winter.

The Beginning

Stimulated by our great master gland, the pituitary, menstrual life sputters and starts as little girls begin to become young women. The rose buds as follows:

In about the ninth year of a girl's life the pituitary gland begins to awaken both ovaries by emitting two powerful hormones—*FSH (follicle stimulating hormone)* and *LH (luteinizing hormone)*.

FSH stimulates one or more of the thousands of immature eggs (follicles) in the ovaries to begin a maturation cycle. Although it may be several years before *ovulation,* the process in which one maturing egg ruptures from the ovarian capsule and follows its course, FSH induces the maturing eggs to begin to secrete *estrogen,* the primary female hormone. Mainly under the influence of estrogen, genital maturation begins. This maturation includes growth and development of the secondary sexual apparatus, such as the breasts and thighs, and the primary apparatus, which includes the vagina along with the uterus and its lining, the *endometrium.* The endometrium begins to undergo cyclical changes and menstruation begins (menarche) even before regular ovulation takes place.

LH sooner or later forces *ovulation* (see glossary) to take place, and a physiological cyst called the *corpus luteum* forms where ovulation has occurred. This cyst secretes the hormone *progesterone,* which, among many other things, prepares the endometrium (during a 14-day term) for a fertilized egg. If none arrives, the corpus luteum shrinks and stops making progesterone, the endometrium withers and menstruation (menses) occurs. Ovulation begins 14 days after the onset of the last menstrual period. And so it goes, more or less regularly, every 28 days, unless pregnancy intervenes. If it does, the corpus luteum lives on, continuing to make the progesterone which, in turn, continues to nurture the endometrium, and so menstruation does not take place. Thus, the very first sign of pregnancy. No period.

Unless interrupted by pregnancy or some other phenomenon, this regular cycle continues until the menopause. There are many problems associated with menstruation. Not all of them are dealt with in this handbook. Some, however, are related to the menopause and thus become our problems, and they will have their moment with us.

The Menopause

The menopause is likely to come upon you as you approach your middle forties—but before we get into it here, some terms need to be defined.

Menopause. This is what our book is all about—but few people can agree upon what the menopause actually is. *MPX* is a medical abbreviation for "menopause," and we will use it often. The word was coined by a Frenchman from Greek words meaning, roughly, end of monthlies. But in modern usage it has become synonymous with all the events that take place as the ovaries cease to function. Thus, the interruption, irregularity or cessation of periods and the attendant emotional and physical changes—some of which (bone calcium loss, for instance) continue to be an influence for the remainder of life—are all considered to be "menopausal" and part of the total "menopausal complex." And that is the way menopause will be considered in our handbook—the beginning of the great adventure.

Climacteric. This term includes all the emotional and physical changes that take place as ovarian function diminishes—but it does not necessarily include the physical cessation of menstrual periods. Thus, the climacteric embraces such symptoms as flushes, night sweats, insomnia, emotional instability, depression, fatigue, forgetfulness, palpitations and so forth. The climacteric ceases—by definition—in a few years. The *change of life* might be considered synonymous with the climacteric.

Perimenopause. The years that immediately precede the menopause are called the perimenopause (PeriMPX). At this time the *premenstrual syndrome* (described below) is likely to be exaggerated. Moreover, even while menstruation remains reasonably regular, menopausal symptoms often are felt. Thus, flushes, night sweats, palpitations, emotional instability, forgetfulness and more are not uncommon at this time and will accelerate as the menopause moves along.

Postmenopause. From the time that ovarian function ceases more or less completely (but never quite completely, unless the ovaries are diseased or removed surgically), women enter their postmenopausal life. Without hormone replacement, the postmenopausal (PMPX) years usually consist of a continuous gradual decline in physical and emotional function.

Premature (early) menopause. When a woman's ovarian function declines early in life—anytime before she reaches the age of forty—a premature menopause exists. It may be temporary (because of illness, strenuous physical activity, stress, etc.) or permanent (resulting from removal of the ovaries, a familial or autoimmune disorder or destructive ovarian disease). Whether temporary or permanent, typical menopausal symptoms occur.

Premenstrual syndrome (PMS). Existing since the beginning of time but only recently legitimized, this condition is characterized by certain emotional and physical changes that precede each menstruation by a few days to a week. Commonly, there is retention of fluid (swelling, edema), breast tenderness, headaches, irritability, emotional instability, depression, fatigue, lassitude, insomnia and considerably more. Many women aptly refer to this distressing cycle of events as a Jekyll-Hyde existence. The PMS tends to deepen and to last longer as the perimenopause deepens and the menopause approaches.

As a general pattern, ovarian function begins to decline somewhere between forty-five and fifty. The ovaries run out of eggs that are capable of maturation and hormone production and, as a result, the pituitary gland, recognizing the ovarian decline, emits exceedingly high levels of FSH to try to get the ovaries' attention. It doesn't work—at least not for long—and ovarian function, ovulation and hormone production all diminish.

The loss of ovarian progesterone and then estrogen leaves the endometrium without adequate nourishment, and so menstruation becomes erratic and eventually ceases.

The loss of *progesterone* causes several changes, including a few problems:

- There *may* be a temporary decrease in premenstrual symptoms.

- Irregular and abnormal periods are much more likely to occur.

- If estrogen secretion continues (even in small amounts) in the absence of progesterone, cancer of the endometrium, and perhaps of the breasts, is more likely to take place down the line. As we shall see, small amounts of estrogen may continue to be present and function in the body during the postmenopausal years by a variety of mechanisms. Without progesterone to complement it in certain tissues, unopposed estrogen can become a serious malignant irritant.

When *significant* regular *estrogen* production ceases, for whatever reason, very important bodily changes are set in motion:

- The endometrium ceases to grow; it becomes *atrophic* (begins to waste away).

- The uterus begins to shrivel, ending up one-half its active size.

- The vagina also undergoes aging changes. First, its lining skin becomes thin and dry, and loses elasticity and resiliency. The skin appears to be shiny or waxy. Infections are more likely to take place and sexual pain is common. Lubrication is absent.

• Like the vagina, the external genitalia (vulva) become thin, waxy and more subject to irritation and diseases. Lubricating glands stop secreting and the skin is therefore more likely to crack when stretched or irritated. In time, the clitoris may become encased in thinning skin, becoming less accessible and responding more slowly—or not at all—to sexual stimulation.

• During the decline in estrogen production, breast tenderness may temporarily increase. Eventually the breasts wither as glandular tissue becomes inactive.

• Generally, all body skin becomes thin and dry. Thus, wrinkling increases and superficial blood vessels appear more prominently. Often the skin darkens, and brown aging spots appear along with dark hair.

• In the absence of estrogen, bone loss accelerates; susceptible women can lose as much as 2 percent of their bone mass each year, producing in time *osteoporosis,* which now destroys more American women than cancer of the uterus and breast *combined.*

• Without estrogen, arteriosclerosis hastens to clog important arteries. This degenerative change is accelerated in the presence of nicotine and excess blood lipids (fats). Thus, postmenopausal women begin to catch up to men in the rates of heart attacks and strokes. At the present time, cardiovascular disease destroys more women than all other conditions COMBINED! It has become the primary reason for longterm HRT (hormone replacement therapy). See Chapter Nine.

- Vasomotor responses in the brain affect the diameter of various blood vessels and are responsible for the "puffs of heat" that plague almost all menopausal women to varying degrees at some time or another. Without hormone replacement, flushes and sweats often persist for years.

- Much as with the premenstrual syndrome, depression, emotional instability, irritability, fatigue, lassitude and insomnia, and more, regularly accompany the other symptoms of estrogen deprivation at the menopause.

- Significant sexual problems may be manifested at this stage and become progressively more severe as time goes on. Structurally, as we have seen, the vagina and vulva become thin and dry, prone to infection and likely to make intercourse painful. Moreover, sexual stimulation will not induce natural lubrication. The time it takes to reach orgasm is prolonged, and orgasm may eventually not be achieved at all. Finally, sexual drive is often reduced or evaporates.

All the above changes do take place as estrogen departs—some to greater degrees than others—depending upon a number of circumstances. These categories of estrogen deprivation will all be dealt with as this handbook proceeds. One conclusion from all this, however, is inescapable: The menopause is a hormone deficiency disorder with massive medical and social implications. And it has been neglected too long.

𝒞 Pause and Reflect

During her entire lifetime, a woman produces no more than one-fifth of an ounce of estrogen and progesterone—roughly 6 grams—or the amount of sugar you would put in your morning coffee. Talk about a concentrated sweetener!

All ovarian hormones are manufactured within the body from cholesterol—cholesterol that comes either from food intake or from synthesis within the liver. They are called *steroid* hormones (from the Greek *stereos,* meaning "solid") because, although they are members of the vast alcohol family, they will crystallize solid instead of evaporating. Structurally, they are all nearly identical, but, of course, physiologically they are marvelously unique from one another and in their effects upon the body. Incidentally, the male hormone testosterone is a member of the same steroid family, and almost identical to estrogen except that it has one molecule of water tacked on in an odd location. What a difference a little drink can make!

———————

Lydia Bronte, Director of Carnegie Foundation's Aging Society project, was quoted recently as describing a new maturing age between fifty and seventy-five. Almost imperceptibly, this new stage of adult life has been developing and instead of being a time of decline and death, as it has been historically, it is now a new prime of life. Quoting her directly:

> *Age 65 is no longer a real watershed in physical and mental vigor. An underground and undocumented phenomenon is occurring. People in this age group are already pioneering new lifestyles and new patterns, with no previous models to guide them. They are a priceless resource for society.*

———————

Where did the word "menopause" come from? I am going to tell you, and not only that—I am myself going to translate the two paragraphs of the dissertation given by Professor Gardanne (in Paris, 1812) in which he coined the word. This dissertation was where that word was first actually used.

Forgive my French.

The menstrual cessation has received many names: some calling it "the critical epoch," cessation of the monthly or regulars, others describing it as the disappearance of regulars, others as the disappearance of menses, the retreat of age, decline of age, winter of women, death of sex, the critical time, etc. Finally, one is lost in the profusion of names.

The word "menopause" (ménépausie), I believe, expresses perfectly the ideas that one attaches to these diverse events; "menopause" is composed of two Greek words— "month" and "terminate."

And there you have it.

Of all the people in the world who *ever* lived past sixty-five years of age, two thirds are alive today! Moreover, it is estimated that 35,000 Americans living today will reach their one hundredth birthday! (*Journal of the American Medical Association*, 267; 624, 1992.)

2

PREMATURE MENOPAUSE

Things come and go, but not always on schedule. And so it is with normal rhythmic ovarian function. Unlike the cycles of the moon, the sun and the stars in their courses, regular ovarian function from the very onset is neither immutable, unshakable or totally predictable. Thus ovarian function may cease well before the expected forty-fifth year. And such a halt may signal temporary ovarian failure (TOF) or premature (and permanent) ovarian failure (POF).

Temporary Ovarian Failure

Temporary ovarian failure (TOF), like POF, begins with failure to ovulate (and thus no production of progesterone—remember?) and generally progresses until little or no ovarian hormone production exists at all. Thus, both estrogen and progesterone are absent. TOF implies that recovery can and does occur—generally with the elimination or control of the inciting cause or causes.

What Causes Temporary Ovarian Failure?

Temporary ovarian failure may result from any of the following causes:

- *Stress.* Events or conditions that rob the body of internal homeostasis, or balance, very quickly affect the pituitary/ovary relationship and cause the ovaries to shut down. Stress is the commonest cause of TOF and any source of stress—good (traveling abroad) or bad (loss of a loved one)—can at least temporarily arrest ovarian function. Other common stresses include excessive physical activity (intense athletic training), anorexia, obesity, unemployment and being in love, in arrears or in debt. You may be aware of others.

- *Systemic disorders.* Particularly when they are out of control, systemic disorders can arrest ovarian function until recovery from the particular condition takes place. Thus, diabetes, hypertension (high blood pressure), anemia and other serious generalized disorders will produce TOF and amenorrhea (absence of menstruation). Chemotherapy and radiation for cancer have a similar depressive ovarian effect—and one that is not always temporary. Similarly, acute health problems such as serious surgery or infections often induce short-term TOF. If elevated, *prolactin,* a pituitary hormone, can also interrupt menstruation until the pituitary disorder responsible for its elevation is corrected. Ovulation, of course, ceases with this disorder. Certain disorders of the thyroid and adrenal glands can interrupt ovarian function until such disorders can be controlled.

- *Ovarian disease.* Certain ovarian tumors and infections will temporarily suppress normal ovarian function. As an example, an unusual masculinizing tumor of the ovaries usually first declares itself by bringing an end to menstruation.

And there are others; they must all, of course, be successfully treated before ovarian function may resume.

- *Destructive habits.* The use of tobacco, alcohol and drugs
  and certain abnormal eating habits (bulimia, anorexia and
  malnutrition) all have a marked effect on ovarian activity
  and all can induce TOF and amenorrhea.

- *Birth control pills.* Oral contraceptives suppress ovulation
  and largely supplant ovarian function. When oral contraceptives are discontinued, the ovaries, shackled for so
  long, may hesitate before taking their first step toward re-
  gaining normal function. Once in a while, they need help.

The Diagnosis of Temporary Ovarian Failure

How is TOF diagnosed? Although it may seem too obvious to
mention, pregnancy must first be ruled out when a period—or a
number of periods—are missed. A surprising number of unnecessary tests have been ordered due to this blind spot or diagnostic oversight. When pregnancy is confirmed by examination
or laboratory testing, a new adventure begins somewhere else.

After pregnancy has been eliminated as a possible cause, a
complete physical examination and regular laboratory studies
are in order. Thus, any systemic disorder that might contribute
to the ovarian failure can be identified. A *provocative* or *challenge
progesterone test* is the most usual next step. A fixed dose of progesterone is administered either by mouth for seven days or by a
single injection. Menstrual bleeding will follow within a few days
or a few weeks *if* the ovaries have been secreting enough estrogen to prime the endometrium; the externally supplied progesterone completes the endometrial maturation and produces a
period.

If a period *does* follow this challenge, we know that the endometrium is working and will respond to adequate hormone stim-

ulation. It is not the cause of the menstrual cessation. We also know that the ovaries are failing to ovulate but are still producing estrogen. Failure is not complete.

If menstruation does not respond to the challenge, we then supply both estrogen and progesterone in a cyclic manner. A menstrual response following this degree of stimulation tells us that the endometrium is healthy, needing only hormone food for growth, and that ovarian failure is complete, since neither estrogen nor progesterone is being secreted.

Now we have established that ovarian failure exists. Is it temporary or permanent? Is it a disorder of the ovaries themselves (primary) or is it from an outside source (secondary)?

More testing is now necessary. Studies of pituitary, adrenal and thyroid gland function are all very relevant. The pituitary studies test FSH, LH and prolactin levels at the very least. Adrenal gland disorders that can interrupt menstruation are not uncommon and involve the abnormal production of both *cortisone* and certain other adrenal hormones with masculinizing characteristics; these hormone levels are tested as well. Tests are also taken to determine if increased or decreased thyroid functions have halted menses. Certain other thyroid (and adrenal, for that matter) tests may determine the presence of autoimmune disorders that also attack the ovaries. See Premature Ovarian Failure, beginning on page 15.

Further observations and studies are necessary to eliminate systemic disorders that may be working their will upon the ovaries. A genetic history and chromosomal studies may be indicated.

Finally, biopsy of the ovaries may have to be done under direct visualization—usually by out-patient laparascopic techniques. The tissue thus obtained is submitted for tissue and molecular genetic studies. Such studies will help determine absolute ovarian function and capabilities.

By following the above outline (and there are many variations to this approach that are employed in different clinics), we can determine whether the ovarian failure is temporary or permanent and proceed with proper care. Let me hasten to say that many times a patient experiences menstrual cessation and the cause is so clear at that time that no intensive workup is indicated. Thus, an otherwise healthy 25-year-old woman in the throes of a difficult divorce, living on cigarettes and coffee, not menstruating and not pregnant, needs our help and not our workup. Menstruation will follow when she is through her troubled time. If it doesn't, then a study can be considered, but it is seldom necessary.

The Treatment of Temporary Ovarian Failure

The management of temporary ovarian failure is easy to outline. First, the doctor and patient must treat the cause, which may not be as simple as it sounds. Nevertheless, treatment should be directed toward the elimination of the offending cause. All the culprits described earlier will generally, sooner or later, yield to appropriate treatment and allow the ovaries to go about their normal business.

Second, *hormone replacement therapy (HRT)* may be necessary. The use of supplemental hormones during this period of temporary failure is generally indicated (unless the failure is extremely short-lived). HRT is important because symptoms of estrogen depletion—including flushes, insomnia and fatigue— are usually present and unpleasant; significant bone loss takes place in prolonged estrogen deprivation at any age; and the endometrium needs regular stimulation to keep it healthy.

HRT may consist of oral contraceptives or other estrogen-progesterone combinations (when oral contraceptives are contraindicated).

Premature Ovarian Failure

Premature ovarian failure (POF) is, by our definition, permanent and complete and represents or, indeed actually is, a premature menopause. It happens before the fortieth year and includes all the symptoms of estrogen deprivation: irregular, delayed menses followed by total cessation of periods; flushes; night sweats; insomnia; fatigue; emotional instability; vaginal dryness and more.

POF involves about 5 percent of all women under forty and is generally preceded by several years of irregular, delayed menses. For these women, the onset of puberty is generally normal but breast development may be depressed. Of the 5 percent of women involved, a third who enter this state of POF have never conceived and about one in ten has a family history of POF.

What Causes Premature Ovarian Failure?

Genetic abnormalities are associated with 18 percent of all premature ovarian failure. Both abnormal sex chromosomes and abnormal regular chromosomes (autosomes) may induce a premature menopause. Women with POF caused by genetic abnormalities are usually short of stature, have a family history of POF, and have other congenital abnormalities that further assist in their clinical identification. Chromosome cultures may clearly identify this problem, but ovarian cell cultures may be necessary in a "mosaic" individual (one who has inherited and carries two distinct cell lines that may not be detected by routine genetic culturing). Thus, blood chromosome cultures may be normal but ovarian chromosome cultures may not.

Autoimmune disorders are responsible for at least 12 percent of all premature ovarian failure. Under these circumstances the body builds self-destructive antibodies to its own glandular system, causing a sort of polyglandular suicide. These antibodies, which are usually directed against the adrenal and thyroid glands, can also be detected, though only with considerable difficulty. Not every clinic can do it.

Defects in ovarian metabolism and function probably account for 12 percent of all POF. In this broad dysfunction, all of the proper eggs are present and in order but due to metabolic failure that is poorly understood, maturation does not take place and hormone secretion fails.

Severe ovarian damage from radiation, chemotherapy and infection, along with, of course, surgical removal of the ovaries, eliminates all function associated with these glands. Moreover, there is evidence that, even conserving the ovaries while removing the uterus, permanent ovarian failure may be hastened by several years. Ovarian damage accounts for 40 percent of all POF.

Acquired defects caused by viral disorders (mumps, for instance) particularly at the time of puberty, along with certain other systemic infections, are sometimes responsible for POF in later years. These defects account for 8 percent of POF.

All the remaining causes of POF—which account for about 10 percent of the total cases—are grouped in the unknown category. As time goes by, this category diminishes in size but will probably always exist.

The Diagnosis of Premature Ovarian Failure

A great number of cases of premature ovarian failure can be identified through a medical history. A history of familial and inherited disorders, or of ovarian damage or removal, or of radiation or chemotherapy or of many other causes can be elicited just by talking to the patient. Confirmatory evidence is easy to obtain.

Temporary ovarian failure must be eliminated by the procedures listed above.

Chromosome culturing and autoimmune testing can be done in appropriate clinical settings where such procedures are available. When they are not immediately available, blood specimens drawn in any office can generally be transferred to research laboratories capable of providing exact results in a reasonable period of time. Not always, though, at a reasonable price!

Ovarian biopsy may provide the definitive answer. Proper ovarian sampling taken directly and in adequate amounts will establish whether there is any finite pattern of ovarian life expectancy. The absence of follicles capable of maturation clearly indicates that ovarian function has permanently ceased.

The Treatment of Premature Ovarian Failure

Hormone replacement therapy is very important and should be instituted early. Early treatment can prevent osteoporosis, delay arteriosclerosis, prevent involution and atrophy of the sexual system and sexual drive and allay early menopausal symptoms.

These needs all will be clearly explained as we move on. Along with HRT it is important to carry out all the other programs—diet, exercise, lifestyle and the like—that can be found in this book.

ℰ Pause and Reflect

By the twentieth week of gestation, a female fetus has 6 to 7 million immature eggs in her ovaries—the most she will ever have. At birth, about 1 million eggs remain, and at puberty, only 300,000 are left. Of these, only about 300 will mature and undergo ovulation during a normal lifetime. Thus 99.9 percent of all the eggs are lost along the way!

How the 300 eggs that will be released from the ovaries are awakened and committed to ovulation is not yet fully understood. The process is, however, relentless, and continues on whether ovulation is suppressed (by birth control pills, for instance) or not. Any process that diminishes the number of available immature follicles at puberty or hastens their death will hasten premature ovarian failure.

Recent studies of rodents have revealed some reproductive aging secrets. In one study, a group of young rats had their ovaries surgically removed. When the rats grew old, they had fresh young ovaries implanted and the rats began regular cyclic activity just as youngsters would! This piece of research might lead to techniques that allow human ovarian activity to be suspended— for whatever reason—and reactivated in later years. So can one have a baby at sixty? I doubt it. But important uses of such research may come in time. And our pool of knowledge grows—as does our indebtedness to fragile little animals.

Forty years ago two scientists first reported the double helix structure of DNA—the basic building blocks of genes, chromosomes and us. This discovery has led to startling advances in molecular genetic biology and in the practice of medicine.

- Diagnosis of genetic disorders has become exceedingly accurate.

- There is increasing understanding of the genetic basis of many common disorders—for example, cancer.

- Using recombinant genetic techniques, we will eventually eliminate the risks involved by using our present human pooled material.

- Creative genetic engineering will eliminate some disorders that we can now only treat supportively—for example, immunodeficiency diseases.

- Genetic engineering may one day allow us to insert genes that can correct a host of inherited conditions. One of them could be a gene to prevent premature ovarian failure.

Interfering with nature? So is immunization, insulin and antibiotics.

3

THE PREMENSTRUAL SYNDROME AND THE PERIMENOPAUSE

As surely as the night follows the day, ovarian decline gradually takes place as the late thirties and early forties unfold. Such a decline is minute and almost not measurable in these early years, but some things do begin to happen.

- The premenstrual syndrome (PMS) that involves many women during their cyclic menstrual years often becomes more intense at this time of life.

- The perimenopause—comprising a few years preceding the full-blown acute menopause—may well produce some vague symptoms of its own.

Let's look at these two.

The Premenstrual Syndrome

(Start by reading in your Bible—Hebrews, 13:8)

You may—quite naturally—still wonder why, in a book dealing mainly with the menopause and postmenopause, I would include a section on PMS. Fair enough. Here are my reasons:

- PMS is associated with cyclic ovarian hormone activity and is not seen before puberty, during pregnancy or after the menopause.

- PMS will continue after a hysterectomy (removal of the uterus) if the ovaries are still active and functioning.

- The disorder seems to intensify as the perimenopause intensifies (see p. 24).

- The symptoms multiply before a period and disappear with the onset of a flow—again indicating a hormone involvement. Female hormones are a big part of our discussion in this book.

Syndrome is a medical term that means a collection of symptoms we don't understand. The premenstrual syndrome has been described in popular books, novels, poems, plays and even in the medical literature since the beginning of recorded history. The condition wasn't given a name until 1953 and even after being named was generally disregarded by the healing profession until very recently—even though at least half of all women are troubled by it and as many as 10 percent are afflicted seriously enough to suffer real interference with their social and work responsibilities.

What do we know about it?

- It is real—not psychological—although psychological events play a real role in the disorder.

- It is cyclic—related to the timing of menses flow.

- Extensive biochemical, endocrinological, sociological and psychological studies have failed to reveal the basic cause.

- PMS is considered a legal defense for women in Britain and France, but not yet in the United States.

- There is a considerable "placebo" response. Some 30 to 50 percent of the women under treatment improve on inert pills. This is the real psychological component.

- In our society, PMS is more common among inactive women with stressful lifestyles and improper dietary habits.

Though we don't know the causes of this crippling condition, these are the popular theories that have been proposed and studied.

- Hormones. Despite what I have said about PMS being hormone-related, all attempts to alter the hormone environment in multitudes of studies have failed to come up with a solution. This includes the much-heralded progesterone program so recently in vogue. Remember again, placebo effect.

- Sugar metabolism. Since cravings for sugar are common during PMS, studies of sugar function have been widely explored. No significant changes in blood glucose levels, or insulin or glucose tolerance have been demonstrated.

- Vitamin and mineral deficiency. Vitamin B complex, B6, and various minerals have all failed the statistical significance test.

- Fluid retention. This has been a popular theory. There is no doubt fluid is retained premenstrually. The theory holds that fluid retained in the brain and breasts produces most of the PMS symptoms. Removal of the fluid with diuretics, however, only relieves fluid-related symptoms. It is not the answer.

- Prostoglandins (body substances known to cause menses cramping) and endorphins (other body substances involved in pain control and other complex body functions) are now being studied as the possible underlying agents producing PMS. Nothing substantial has turned up. Yet.

Knowing as little as we do about your PMS, how can we treat the swelling, fluid retention, tender breasts, headaches, bloating, anxiety, irritability, restlessness, depression, hostility, food cravings and more that will apparently be with you today and forever?

First, it is important to be reasonably sure that PMS is what we are facing. Usually a conscientious personal diary of symptoms kept over a few months will reveal a great deal and allow the diagnosis to be confirmed or discarded. There are no laboratory studies of any help whatsoever.

When the diagnosis is established, the specific symptoms are isolated and treated individually.

- Fluid retention is managed by the appropriate water pills (diuretics) and dietary restrictions.

- Emotional symptoms are treated with a variety of short-term antidepressants or anxiolytic drugs. These drugs change so fast that any named now will be outdated by the time you read this. Better ones keep coming. Your doctor should know which one is best for you.

- Although there is no absolute proof that diet is involved, women who eat nutritionally well and avoid excess salt, sugar, caffeine and chocolate at this time seem to do much better. But that is also true anytime!

- Sleep deprivation is very helpful when emotional complaints are significant—particularly depression. Moreover, increased exposure to light is of great value here—whether the light be from the sun or from an artificial source.

- Learn to cope, resolve conflicts at other times and avoid confrontation during PMS. Make it your dodging time.

The Perimenopause

Just as with PMS, the perimenopause does not disturb all women and often goes by unnoticed. You should simply wait and see what unfolds as your own life moves forward. So, the first observation is—don't look for anything. There may be nothing.

Second, so ingrained is the double standard of aging that it can hardly fail to shake the confidence of the most mature, stable and secure woman. Women have to face not only what the menopause itself actually brings to them, but they must also face what cultures have added to it. As a result of all this interplay, significant psychological storms may now gather strength. It is important to keep these cultural factors in mind as you near the menopause.

You will remember that ovarian function is finite and that the ovaries are organs with a limited active life cycle. Although there are hundreds of thousands of immature follicles in each ovary, only a few hundred in a lifetime can ripen into mature eggs that are capable of being ovulated and fertilized. Moreover, if these eggs are not spent during the reproductive years, they cannot be saved and spent later.

As the ovaries age and the number of capable follicles diminishes, the pituitary gland signals the ovaries (with FSH, the follicle stimulating hormone) to get back to work. Alas, it is of little avail and gradually inferior follicles are stimulated. These marginal follicles produce estrogen as the eggs struggle to mature, but the eggs are incapable of undergoing ovulation. Thus, no progesterone is released and cyclic menstrual bleeding will, as a result, inevitably change. Moreover, the amount of estrogen produced in each cycle will gradually decline, so symptoms of estrogen deficiency will begin to appear. Sometime during this endocrine conflict, the perimenopause makes its appearance.

Depending largely upon the rate of ovarian decline, the perimenopause begins to be felt in the early forties, although women with exceedingly active and healthy ovaries may not experience the PeriMPX until their middle or late forties. Whenever it occurs, it precedes the menopause by two or three years and flows directly into it.

One of the most noticeable changes of the perimenopause involves menstruation. Because progesterone is no longer being secreted, the menstrual flow is liable to be considerably different. Estrogen alone cannot produce a normal endometrium capable of producing a normal period. Bleeding will, in some way, be different during the PeriMPX. Such alterations may be minor— bleeding may be slightly more irregular, somewhat shorter, or somewhat longer—and sometimes prolonged and heavy periods may be the order of the day.

Although bleeding irregularities and problems may arise in the PeriMPX as it leads into the MPX, a number of women have noted that menstruation can cease abruptly with no prior warnings. And unless hormone replacement is instituted, these women never menstruate again. Yet no matter what the pattern, the perimenopause usually involves some menstrual change.

Symptoms of the Perimenopause

Vague symptoms may appear at the start of the PeriMPX, signaling the beginning of ovarian failure. Fatigue, which is recorded in 75 percent of all women at this time, is probably the commonest companion of the perimenopause. Although fatigue is a symptom of many other disorders, its almost unfailing appearance is a common characteristic of the PeriMPX.

Emotional changes—particularly if PMS problems have been present—accelerate at this time. Insomnia (which may contribute to fatigue), depression (which may do the same thing) and irritability are common pitfalls. All of these symptoms, including fatigue, are variable and intermittent. They come and go and are not necessarily cyclic or related to the menstrual cycle.

The Diagnosis of the Perimenopause

There is no known diagnostic sign to assist with the identification of the PeriMPX. Although blood FSH levels may be elevated, they bear no relationship to the symptoms of the PeriMPX. The levels of estrogen and progesterone change so imperceptibly that their measurement is of no use (until progesterone disappears altogether as ovulation ceases). The sensitivity of organs targeted by estrogen and progesterone—the uterus, the breasts, the skin and the vagina—changes as well, but again the change is too slight to be of use in diagnosis. Insidious changes also begin to take place in bone density and in the blood vessels, but these changes occur without symptoms and are almost impossible to measure clinically.

It is clear, and has been said many times before, that not *all* women need or want any help at this time. Minimal or nonexistent symptoms require no supportive therapy by physicians. Nevertheless, regular gynecological examinations and consultations are important for all perimenopausal women, symptoms or not. Seemingly trifling problems that may arise at this time can, if neglected, ignite into crippling disorders in later years.

Annual or semiannual examinations and consultations are the cornerstone of proper PeriMPX management. The frequency of these visits depends upon your level of symptoms and complications.

Examinations should be preceded by a problem-oriented consultation. Such talks should be conducted with both participants sitting up. This has not always been so—as many of you already know. Modern examining equipment and enlightened competitive gynecologists, however, have largely dispelled the unequal environment.

You should have a Papanicolaou (Pap) smear done at least once a year, whether or not a hysterectomy has previously been performed. (See page 50.) Your doctor should take your blood pressure, record your height and weight and do a urinalysis and a blood count.

Less frequent, but equally important, are tests of the blood fats—cholesterol, triglycerides and others—plus regular mammograms and a baseline one-time bone density test. A hormone smear is also recommended.

The Treatment of the Perimenopause

Your postexamination consultation should include a discussion of any positive findings and help reinforce the significant aspects of your lifestyle—diet and exercise, along with drug, nicotine and alcohol control. In addition, you should discuss the possible need for calcium and vitamin D supplements as well as for hormone replacement therapy.

If sufficient abnormal bleeding or subjective symptoms are present and HRT is indicated, certain oral contraceptives are perfect for the job. Here are some things about the oral contraceptive pill, or OC, that you might want to know:

- OCs cannot be used under any circumstances for women who smoke. A woman who is addicted to tobacco at this time in her life subjects herself to a tenfold increase in death from heart disease if she uses OCs. Most nonsmokers may, however, use OCs with safety. The pill will resolve the nonsmoker's perimenopausal problems and keep her from conceiving (pregnancy is a condition that, at this time in a woman's life, involves much greater risks than does the pill).

- Oral contraceptives do not increase the risk of gallbladder disease. Instead, they offer protection against certain pelvic infections and may also protect against anemia from excessive menstrual blood loss.

- There is increasing evidence that OCs protect the breasts, the ovaries and the lining of the uterus from cancer, even for years after the OCs have been discontinued.

For these and other reasons, the birth control pill may be an ideal agent in managing the perimenopause. Some general medical problems (high blood pressure, for instance) may mitigate this fact. Your gynecologist will best advise you.

Because all the topics covered in a physical examination and consultation are so very important, they will be discussed in greater detail in the chapters that follow.

ℰ Pause and Reflect

According to the Census Bureau in Washington, there will be 6.2 billion people on earth by the year 2000. In comparison, there were 3 billion in 1960. Although the United States population will not reproduce as rapidly as that of some Third World countries, there will still be a hefty increase in our population—at a rate of four every second!

Our population mix will change considerably by this century's end. Today's yuppies will be senior citizens by then. The menopausal population will be vastly larger and will continue to be an enlightened coterie with money to burn and the good sense not to burn it.

———————

Another interesting explosion is taking place. Over 6,000 medical articles see print every day. Every day! Right now the body of our scientific information *doubles* every five years, and will soon double every two years. How much of that do you think your doctor can read?

Precious little—and work at the same time. Your doctor has to be helped by computer and other summary services to digest what new information is important to her.

———————

And while we are on the subject of gynecologists—and women—it has been proven that female physicians spend more time with their patients than do their male counterparts. Moreover, in 1986 there were, for the first time, more female than male residents specializing in obstetrics and gynecology. Not only that, the pass rate for certification examination in obstetrics and gynecology was greater for females than males.

In addition, women believe their gynecologists are more honest than anyone other than members of the clergy! More honest than their own husbands! Least honest? Auto mechanics (17 percent), the President (8 percent) and Congress (3 percent).

———————

Women outlive men, but this fact may soon change. Men are not getting healthier; women are catching more of men's problems. Why? Women are increasingly beset by high blood pressure, obesity and diabetes; the incidence of lung cancer in women has risen *600 percent* in the past thirty years, and lung cancer now kills more women than men; more women are involved with alcohol and drugs, as well as with cigarettes, because of changing societal roles and stresses; more women now suffer from suicidal depression; and breast cancer strikes one woman in nine. The greatest insult among all these is smoking.

Our psychiatric brethren have, in their infinite wisdom, decided to add PMS to their litany of emotional disorders. Thus you can find it codified in *The Diagnostic and Statistical Manual of Mental Disorders,* Third Edition, Revised. Not only that—they have given it a newer, bigger and more important name. Get this: "The Luteal Phase Dysphoric Disorder"! No clubs have yet been formed.

Apropos the above message from the psychiatrists, the following statement appeared in the *Journal of the American Medical Association* in June 1891: "Menstrual anomalies make up a sixth part of all the causes of insanity"!

I have often been asked if men had any cyclic hormone changes that could produce within them PMS-like symptoms. The answer, of course, is no—men are that way all the time.

Here are a few more interesting asides about PMS.

- It is but one of seventy health problems that regularly vary with cyclic ovarian activity.

- There are at least eighty different active programs for managing PMS.

- Some observers say they have NEVER seen PMS in female athletes.

Here are some PMS help sources:

- The PMS Self-Help Center
101 First Street, Suite 441
Los Altos, CA 94022
Tel. (415) 964–7268

- PMS HOTLINE: 1–800–222–4PMS

- "PMS"—a booklet distributed by:
Chattem Consumer Products
1715 West 38th Street
Chattanooga, TN 37409

4

THE MENOPAUSE

The vagaries of semantics are nowhere more obvious than with the word "menopause." As already noted in the first chapter, the menopause (MPX) signifies, scientifically, *only the absolute cessation of menses*. At least, that is the present-day definition of the menopause. Yet the word "menopause," as it is popularly used, signifies the whole panorama of events and symptoms that flow from the onset of the MPX and encompasses all that happens in the ensuing several years—both physical and emotional. This includes not only the cessation of periods but the starting of the "change"—of flushes and sweats and insomnia and fatigue and all the other events that may be waiting in the wings.

But the proper word for this continuum of insults is the *climacteric*. Scientists, gynecologists, endocrinologists and everyone else involved in menopausal management use this word to describe all the events that we are talking about and that you are struggling with. In fact, the leading "change of life" clinics in this country were once called "climacteric clinics." I tried running one, too. We all ended up seeing patients with sexual problems! The clinics have mainly been renamed.

These definitions are clearly established in medical literature. You and I, however, will continue to call all the things that are happening at the time of your life when menstruation ceases and *shortly* thereafter "the menopause (MPX)," and will call those things that follow these tumultuous events and last forever "the postmenopause (PMPX)."

Our final definition of the menopause, then, is the cessation of natural menstruation and the events (symptoms) that shortly precede and follow it.

Having resolved the issue of terms—at least to our satisfaction—it is safe to move on.

Moving on is what the menopause is all about. You are already aware that those things that are happening when menstruation ceases *do not* represent an abrupt change in function or a sudden decline in body function.

Slowly, but inexorably, ovarian function continues to subside as certain landmark events take place. As we noted earlier, ovulation ceases, and with it the production and secretion of progesterone. Estrogen secretion from the ovaries declines gradually until not enough is produced to support and bring forth a menstrual flow.

It is clear that if the ovaries have been surgically removed or if ovarian function has been destroyed by disease, there follows an abrupt and complete cessation of both estrogen and progesterone production. This event may evoke profound bodily changes that we will also look at as we move along.

Let's note here that the ovaries will continue to make *some* estrogen and estrogen-like substances, probably throughout your entire life, although this is a variable phenomenon. Many estrogen-like substances that the ovary produces at this time have masculinizing elements in their structure. Such elements may account for an increase in sex drive in certain postmenopausal women and for certain masculinizing tendencies, such as an increase in facial hair, that these women may exhibit.

There are two basic ovarian estrogens: estrone (E1) and estradiol (E2).

The production of E1 and E2 parallel one another during normal menstrual life as they are both excreted by maturing follicles. E2 is a more powerful estrogen than E1. Before the menopause, a small amount of E1 is made from a circulating male-like hormone called androstenedione. This conversion takes place in fatty tissues. After the menopause, more androstenedione (95 percent of which is made in the adrenal gland and 5 percent of which is produced in the ovaries) is converted to E1 in fatty tissue. This fact accounts for *some* of the postmenopause estrogen in heavy women. Moreover, increasing postmenopausal dominance of androstenedione, as we have seen, produces masculine-like tendencies in some older women—facial hair growth and breast atrophy—and even increased sex drive.

Since E2 is primarily the product of the developing follicle, its level drops dramatically at the menopause. Thereafter it is produced in small amounts by conversion of E1 in target organs such as the breasts.

You will see as our story unfolds how these variable hormone factors can affect the outcome of the menopausal treatment.

When Does the Menopause Occur?

We have already noted that menstruation may cease when a woman is anywhere between forty-five and fifty years of age. This has been historically true. In addition:

- There are ethnic variations in menopausal onset but the studies reporting such differences are poorly controlled for other variables such as health, nutrition and climate.

- Neither the age at which menstruation begins nor family history has any influence on the time of menopause.

- Thin women, malnourished women and women who smoke all have a significantly earlier menopause.

- The effect of marital status and family size upon entry into menopause is hotly debated and unsettled. A single recent study indicates that women who have sustained repeated abortions may have an earlier menopause.

- Higher altitudes produce an earlier menopause.

- The effect of long-term birth control pill usage upon menopausal onset is, as yet, unknown.

What Is the Menopause Like?

The menopause comprises many symptoms. Not every woman experiences all of them, and not all symptoms are felt with equal depth. Thus flushes may be incapacitating to some, but only minor nuisances to others. Listed below are the major symptoms associated with the menopause.

Hot Flashes (Flushes) and Night Sweats

Typically a flush starts deep within the chest, as intense heat, and flows upward and outward through the shoulders, neck and head. It is followed by some degree of sweating. The sufferer feels this heat and is aware, rightly or wrongly, that everyone can see the flush. Such episodes end in a few moments and can recur every few minutes or hours, depending upon a number of circumstances. Often, there follows a short period of faintness or weakness.

What Produces a Hot Flush?

Here, with some simplification, is the actual sequence of physiological events in a typical hot flush cycle. Diminished estrogen levels irritate certain sensitive neuroreceptors in the base of the brain. These neuroreceptors in turn signal peripheral blood vessels in the upper body to dilate (expand). We are now just a few minutes away from a flush.

Gradually the dilated blood vessels heat up the skin and as that happens, a flush unfolds. While skin temperature is rising during the several minutes of a flush, body core temperature begins to drop a few degrees. This cooling effect is heightened because newly formed perspiration evaporates from the skin. Chills may now follow this double cooling phenomenon.

As a result of body cooling, the hormone adrenalin begins to circulate; the adrenal gland is invoking its "involuntary fight or flight" response. Peripheral blood vessels constrict and the flush ends. Five minutes have elapsed.

Some other things happen during a flush. Oxygen consumption increases. So does the pulse rate. Electrocardiograph recordings reveal fluctuations in heartbeat outside normal limits, but clearly without harmful effect.

Although flushes are the most common symptom of the menopause, their intensity and occurrence rate varies greatly from one woman to another. Nevertheless, 85 percent of all menopausal women experience flushes for over a year and up to 50 percent for over five years.

Night sweats are essentially the same as the daytime flushing phenomenon, but work their magic during normal sleep. Heat generated by the flush that occurs while you are sleeping makes you kick off your sheets and blankets; this subconscious baring of the flesh is naturally followed by body coolness from evaporating sweat. Thus the classic nocturnal "cold sweat."

External stimuli can initiate a hot flush. Thus, a doorbell

ring, a sudden auto stop, a phone call from your gynecologist, a new perfume scent—any number of things can "turn up the heat." Dreams can also cause night sweats.

Unlike many of the serious long-term consequences of the MPX (osteoporosis, for instance), flushes and sweats gradually diminish and disappear after a variable number of years. Hormone replacement therapy completely obliterates flushes and sweats.

Insomnia

"Think in the morning. Act in the noon. Eat in the evening. Sleep in the night."

Good advice for all times, but sleep may be denied those of you struggling with the menopause. Insomnia becomes a companion almost as faithful as flushes. And there are several reasons why this is so.

A hot flush brings wakefulness, and the cold sweat that follows each flush requires the readjustment of sheets, covers, coverlets, quilts, pillows, your nightgown and your bedfellow. And when that's all over with, you're about 10,000 behind on the sheep count. Even if sleep comes again, there is another night sweat waiting close by in the wings. And it all starts again.

Depression is clearly associated with the menopause and it involves a significant number of menopausal women. Since early-morning wakefulness is a common companion of depression it may therefore involve MPX women, even when night sweats do not.

Other menopausal associates—irritability, heart palpitations and formications (numb, itchy or irritable extremities)—can all contribute to restless nights.

Clearly, there is an abundance of reasons why you should not sleep well during the MPX—and the lack of sound, uninterrupted sleep probably contributes heavily to fatigue. Fortunately, hormone replacement therapy will control almost all menopausal insomnia.

Fatigue

Every once in a while a patient of long standing will arrive for her annual visit and consultation complaining of "fatigue."

Now in her early forties, my patient friend will still have regular periods, no hot flushes or night sweats, excellent health and habits, will sleep well and have no family or work problems, but will be inexplicably exhausted. She gets up in limbo, drags during the day and is ready for the sheets before the six P.M. news is over.

Generally, a complete physical examination and the standard blood work will yield no helpful information. And that is because her "fatigue" is really one of the earliest indications of the MPX, which, as we already know, may be first noted in the perimenopause.

It is important here for the patient and the physician to be certain that there are no physical or emotional causes for the tiredness other than the menopause itself. Sleep must be adequate, sustained and relatively free from interruptions. In addition, nighttime visits to the bathroom need to be recorded since they tend to become more of a constant presence at this time and signal the beginnings of the menopause.

Emotional Problems

Scientists and physicians—both male and female—who have studied the menopause as a career cannot agree upon the psychological content of the menopause and, in many cases, simply state their own convictions. Gynecologists—both male and female—have just now begrudgingly added emotional problems to their lexicon of menopausal symptoms.

No matter what the opinions are or who holds them, one

thing has been clearly proven: Hormone replacement therapy will alleviate most menopausal emotional problems.

Here is a list of the commonest emotional symptoms found in the menopause: depression, irritability, anxiety, insomnia, tension, antisocial behavior, headaches, inability to concentrate, loss of sex drive, nervousness, aggressiveness.

Over half of all menopausal women will experience some (but not all) of these disturbances, and they may last for several years. It is important that they be differentiated from the true psychological illnesses that might well occur coincidentally at this time. Thus a depression may be MPX-related or may be a true and separate entity requiring special treatment. Clearly, such unrelated depressions do not respond to hormone therapy. The same is true of other nonmenopausal-related psychological disorders.

Sexuality

As noted above, the desire for sexual activity often diminishes at this time. This timing may be coincidental since most women's sexual appetite usually—but not always—begins to diminish slowly after the mid-thirties, and the change may become noticeable only in the mid-forties. Yet whatever the reason, loss of sexual drive is common during the menopause.

Other sexual changes become apparent as estrogen secretion diminishes. Erotic stimulation (local or general) fails to produce the usual vaginal lubrication. Time-to-orgasm may be increased, and orgasm may be difficult to achieve. Finally, as the vaginal skin becomes thinner and drier, intercourse becomes more painful and vaginal infections more common.

These changes do not take place instantly at the menopause. They are gradual events that increase in intensity over several years. Women who, somehow, somewhere, continue to make limited amounts of estrogen may exhibit few of these sexual changes until very late in their postmenopausal years. And certain women, because of the increase of male-like hormones in their postmenopausal life, will experience an increase in sexual drive.

The effect of hormone replacement on sexual drive is very complex and will be looked at carefully later on. (See pages 125–28.)

Less Common Menopause Problems

FORMICATIONS. This questionable-sounding word—already mentioned—designates conditions that affect the skin and peripheral tissues. Itchy, numb, tingling arms and legs, fidgety feet, tender joints and so forth are included in this category.

PALPITATIONS. When you become consciously aware of your heartbeat, whether it's fast, slow or irregular, you are experiencing palpitations. Palpitations are generally accompanied by feelings of apprehension and anxiety, but when palpitations are a symptom of the menopause, the condition does not signify harm.

There are other disorders that will produce palpitations—at any time of life—and care must be taken in assigning this symptom to the menopause. On the other hand, simple menopausal palpitations are frequently and falsely diagnosed as heart disorders; both doctors and patients must be aware of this symptom of the menopause and treat it accordingly.

LOSS OF MEMORY (FOR RECENT EVENTS ONLY). You remember your third cousin's birthday but can't remember where you set your drink down. Or you can remember your 1968 income tax payment but can't remember why you just got in the car. Some physicians say that such memory loss comes from an inability to concentrate, but whatever the cause, it is real and it is a nuisance.

Ongoing Problems

It is important to remember that other major events that we have already alluded to continue their march through the menopausal territory. Because of estrogen depletion, bone loss accelerates, arteriosclerosis accelerates, fertility declines and disappears, sexual organs atrophy and skin and breast tissue lose tone and elasticity. These problems will be mentioned again in great detail in our discussion of the postmenopause for, although they start here, they continue to work their will in the years that follow.

How Is the Menopause Diagnosed?

With all these symptoms occurring to one degree or another, what signs are present to help physicians make the diagnosis of menopause? Not many.

After taking the menopausal history, your doctor will proceed to examine you (the components of this exam will be outlined in the next chapter). Such a physical examination reveals few of the vast changes that slowly brought you to the menopause. Everything appears the same as it did one year ago—or five years ago (unless you have some other problems—like excess weight or high blood pressure—that has overtaken you).

What about lab tests? The procedures of real diagnostic help test for blood levels of FSH (elevated) and of estrogen (depressed). As you will recall FSH is secreted by the pituitary gland during reproductive life to stimulate ovarian activity, make an egg mature and produce estrogen. As the ovaries continue to fail the pituitary sends out more FSH to try and revive them. Of course, the FSH jangle is useless at this time because ovarian decline is relentless and irreversible. Circulating estrogen levels also begin to decline—again because of diminishing ovarian activity. These two levels, when detected, strongly support the diagnosis of menopause.

Vaginal hormone smears have been used extensively to measure body estrogen levels and to follow hormone therapy programs. But such smears, while easy to take and read, are not accurate enough to confirm early onset of the menopause—only the advanced menopause—or the results of hormone therapy.

So we are left with little else to help us confirm the diagnosis of menopause save the patient's symptoms and the absence or delay of menses. *And that's plenty.* The symptoms and the absence of menses signify the onset of the menopause. From here we continue our journey into the issues you face in your menopausal years.

ℰ Pause and Reflect

The following facts about estrogen and flushes indicate that hot flashes occur *only* following estrogen withdrawal:

- Women born with congenitally nonfunctional ovaries—thus never making estrogen—also never have hot flashes. Similarly, girls who lose their ovaries because of some catastrophe (like early ovarian malignancy) before menstruation even begins also never have hot flashes.

- Men who have been treated for cancer of the prostate gland with estrogen will have hot flashes when the estrogen is discontinued.

Other problems may produce flush-like episodes:

- People with vasomotor instability blush a lot and have fainting spells at the drop of a thermostat. It is a lifelong characteristic, however.

- High blood pressure, especially when out of control, can often cause recurrent facial flushes. Affecting both men and women, the flushes disappear with appropriate hypertension therapy.

- An overactive (hyperactive) thyroid will often cause flushes which, again, disappear when the thyroid comes under control.

- Emotional problems, including panic attacks, anxiety and depression, also cause flushes.

Do women in other cultures experience the same symptoms at the menopause? The answer to that question is difficult to give because of language barriers, cultural differences and bias on the part of investigators—to name a few of the study problems. Nevertheless, here are some findings:

- 482 Rajput women living in India reported that the menopause was a welcome event noted only because of menstrual cessation. The absence of menstrual flow signaled an incredible elevation of stature for these women. Women were released from a veiled, secluded life in a compound to talk and socialize (even drink) with menfolk. They then became revered as models of wisdom and experience by the younger generation.

- According to one study, Zulu women noted little menopausal symptomology. Another study of Zulu women, however, revealed that many had menopausal problems similar to women in Western societies. Different investigators.

- In all studies of menopausal symptoms, regardless of race, creed, color, social or economic status, one fact stands out: Women who are well-integrated in their environment, who are surrounded by friends and who possess a good social network and have meaningful activities will have less intense menopausal symptoms.

––––––––––

When scientists first suggested using sex hormones for the treatment of depression (in both sexes), they were hooted out of scientific circles, even though the premise was supported by excellent research. Forty years later, however, the data have been "rediscovered," and, indeed, sex hormones now have a valid place in the treatment of many depressions.

––––––––––

If you believe in teleology (the study of final causes, or the philosophy that things have a purposeful end), then you can believe that nature has provided women with a hormonal edge that protects them during the reproductive years. A woman is more resilient to stress and is protected against the harmful consequences of a high-fat diet as long as she has estrogen. When reproduction is beyond her capabilities, her risk of cardiovascular disease matches that of men.

––––––––––

A recent study of right, left and ambihanded women and the menopause revealed some unusual data. The average age at menopause of right-handed women was 47.3; of left-handed women, 42.3; and of ambihanded women, 40.7 years. These are highly significant differences with no clear explanation (Source: *Obstetrics and Gynecology,* 76:1111, 1990).

5

HOW TO SURVIVE—
AND EVEN ENJOY—
THE MENOPAUSE

Getting through childhood could be a very deadly game were it not for some human contrivances. Vaccines, immunization, antibiotics, surgical interventions, burn therapies, leukemia treatment, pasteurized milk, seat harness laws, abuse-monitoring and many more human contrivances have helped make passage through childhood safe. Provided school is not a shooting gallery.

Well, so it is with the menopause. Much is being written about passage through this major lifetime event and safe, positive passage does require some human contrivances and interventions. We are going on now to list the contrivances and interventions that are important to you at this time. All of them will be detailed here or later in your book.

Medical Care

Your primary care physician should be a gynecologist. There are three classes of gynecologists, namely:

- *Generalists*. This category includes gynecologists who conduct a general gynecology practice doing routine female surgical procedures. These physicians also often continue to practice obstetrics.

- *Gynecological oncologists*. These doctors restrict their practice to the management of malignant disorders of the female organs.

- *Infertility gynecologists*. As the name implies, sterility and infertility is the field of interest that engages these gynecologists.

You want a general gynecologist to manage your menopause. The doctors in the other two categories are trying desperately to keep up with their own specialty fields of interest, and as a result they are not as well-versed in the management of the menopause. (Be aware that not all general gynecologists will be interested in treating the menopause; make sure your gynecologist's goals coincide with yours.)

While it is true that almost all physicians can do a routine pelvic, Pap smear and breast examination, it is equally true that hormone replacement therapy has become so complicated that not even all gynecologists are interested in tackling it.

Therefore, I recommend that you seek the care of a competent, caring gynecologist who is interested in menopausal management. There are plenty of them around. If you live in a community that does not have a gynecologist, your own family physician will manage your menopause, checking any problems with a consultant gynecologist as he or she feels necessary.

A successful relationship with your physician requires bilateral openness and willingness to trot out problems on both sides of the desk—or whatever device your consultation takes place over. You, for instance, have to feel free to say that your vagina doesn't lubricate during sex like in the good old days, and your doctor has to feel free to ask you whether your vagina lubricates during sex like it did in the good old days. It is fundamental to your proper care that you tell all you know to be wrong—even if your doctor does not have the good sense to ask for it. Drop at least five of your seven veils.

Since your commitment to your doctor (and your doctor's commitment to you) should be a lengthy one—and hopefully one that has preceded the menopause by some years—you might want to consider your *responsibilities to each other* from now on. Here, for what it's worth, are some of my views.

The Doctor

Listed below are your doctor's responsibilities. He or she should

- Ensure adequate examinations and testing at your regular visits. Arrange for out-of-office examinations (mammograms, blood work, etc.). Properly chart and accumulate data generated by tests and examinations.

- Provide information—with your written permission—to other physicians as you request it, and withhold personal information from all others. Please note that, even if you're not aware of it, you have surrendered this right to privacy to your insurance company and to anyone with whom they wish to share information. That may include other insurance companies, the federal government and your employer's insurance clerk. That's worth remembering.

- Completely disclose benefits and risks when giving—or denying—a certain medication program. "Complete" disclosure means a lot of things. If your doctor suggests surgery at some point, the major risks and benefits need to be laid out for you (although it is impossible to explore every potential risk and benefit). The same is true when discussing hormone replacement therapy.

- Be reasonably available and reasonably current in the areas of his or her responsibility.

- Cover general health problems with you. As doctors, we are very inadequate in this regard. Studies show that we often fail to discuss the elimination of tobacco, moderation of alcohol, use of seat belts, importance of good exercise and dietary habits—the list could go on and on. These things will hurt more of you than the things doctors spend hours talking about. We are as guilty of neglecting to discuss these important health factors as you are of neglecting to practice them.

- Treat you with compassion and understanding. We physicians are healers—not judges, moralists or mechanics.

You

Listed below are your responsibilities. You should

- Keep your appointments and get scheduled tests taken care of as directed. Even if your physician does not send regular reminders through the mail or have his or her staff call you to set up routine visits, you must share some of the responsibility for keeping the relationship going. Somewhere you have a data bank of sorts where you store information and memos. Punch it in.

- Ask questions when you are uncertain about a proposed treatment or procedure or if you don't understand the information you have been given.

- Get a second opinion when you are in real doubt about a proposed therapy plan—be it in surgery, hormone replacement or thermal baths—or about anything your doctor suggests which is major in scope and with which you do not generally agree. Most of the time your doctor will welcome a second opinion, for it usually will confirm his or her position and strengthen your relationship. Also, remember *your* doctor is *someone else's* second opinion. Think about that.

- Comply with your doctor's recommendations. Compliance is one of your major responsibilities. It's yours alone because you have to do the complying. Studies show that, with the possible exception of birth control pills, only about one-third of all clients or patients continue to follow advice or take medications. So follow the dietary, exercise and other general health measures with which you are provided. It's your doctor's responsibility to give such advice. In addition, take medications exactly as outlined, in the amount and at the times prescribed. More is not better and your friend's medicine is probably not right for you. If your medication disagrees with you in any real way, call your doctor.

We have, of course, outlined a perfect doctor/patient relationship—one that exists only between a perfect doctor and a perfect patient in a perfect world. Since that is not the way things are, we must make the best of what we have.

Medical Visits

How often should you visit your gynecologist? Every 6 to 12 months, if there are no complications requiring closer attention.

What is accomplished at this visit? Following a discussion of present symptoms, a regular examination is performed, including a breast and pelvic examination and the measurement of weight, height and blood pressure. In addition, laboratory work is done that includes a Pap smear, urine and blood count and perhaps a hormone smear.

When indicated, a mammogram, a bone density and detailed blood tests may be arranged. Also, a more detailed physical examination may be called for if unusual symptoms are present.

These, in general, are the same procedures that we outlined in the management of the perimenopause. The consultation that follows at this time will, however, deal more specifically with hormone replacement and its management.

Here are some common medical terms that you should know:

PAP SMEAR. This test is named after the Greek-born American anatomist Papanicolaou, who discovered it and persuaded doctors the world over to use it to detect cancer. This smear is taken from the cervix, which is a common site for cancer. The Pap smear can almost always detect the presence of cells destined to cause cancer of the cervix in the future. The smear is of value *only* in screening for malignant and premalignant changes on the cervix or, more rarely, the back of the vagina.

Even with a long history of normal Pap smears, you should have one every two or three years. The sexually transmitted human papilloma virus (HPV) has taken our country by storm and can produce premalignant changes in the cervix at any age. It can do the same thing in the vagina even after a hysterectomy when the cervix is gone. ABSENCE OF THE CERVIX IS NOT

A REASON TO DISCONTINUE PAP SMEARS. Not all physicians will tell you this fact. Finally, if you have had a hysterectomy for a premalignant cervical condition, it is important to have Pap smears taken at very frequent intervals for some years to come.

HORMONE SMEAR. Also known as the *maturation index,* this smear, taken from the vaginal wall, can roughly determine estrogen levels within the body. This is based on the fact that only estrogen can cause the vaginal lining to mature, and thus this amount of estrogen mirrors the levels of estrogen circulating within the body. Estrogen given vaginally as a cream or suppository will, of course, produce a false reading because of its local activity.

BLOOD PROFILES. With automated chemistry, doctors can now easily and relatively cheaply obtain a profile of many body organ systems with one sample of blood. Also known as a *SMAC profile,* a blood profile measures liver and kidney function, blood lipids (or fats, such as cholesterol and triglycerides), sugar, enzymes, electrolytes, thyroid function, serum iron, blood count and often more. Such chemical tests are often important in careful management of the menopause.

Caring for Yourself

While regular contact with your physician is vitally important, there are other things to be done at this time that are also necessary in managing your menopause. Your physician should review much of this substantial material with you at regular visits, and reinforce it from time to time. If your doctor fails to do so, you can learn about it here, even though your own doctor is your best source of information and help.

Diet

Of course, what you eat has been, is now, and will always be of vital importance to you and your well-being.

We are concerned not only with how much we eat but with what we eat. Certain culinary truths prevail:

- One major truth is that the human metabolism—in both men and women—diminishes regularly as we wrestle with the middle years. Thus the "middle-age spread" is a common threat to us all. No matter what, we need fewer and fewer calories each day of our lives. "I don't eat any more than I did before but I still gain!" That won't bake your bread anymore.

- Too much of our diet is fat.

- Weight is a variable depending entirely on what we consume and how much of it is burned as energy.

- Some people can eat more than others and still not gain weight. Conversely, some people can eat less than others and still gain weight.

It is important to follow a diet that is low in fat and one that will not provide you more calories than you need. There are many diet principles that you need to follow; refer to Chapter 6 for a complete discussion of healthful eating. It is an important part of your menopausal and postmenopausal life.

Exercise

It is mind-boggling to contemplate all the devices, the spas, the aerobics classes, the Marquis de Sade running clubs and all the other forced-labor camps that have sprung up to compensate for the physical inactivity that the good life has brought us. The truth is, walking, swimming, cycling or *light*-impact aerobics is all anyone needs to stay healthy.

Exercise is important for cardiovascular fitness and the maintenance of bone strength. It should be regular, enjoyable and productive, though you must be careful not to overexert yourself, as excess exercise can cause damage. Again, a whole section is devoted to proper exercise programs, starting on page 88.

Habits

Our personal habits—as we have been told so many times—are the chains that bind us. Some of our habits are good, and some are bad. Usually a lot are bad. The bad ones have a way of intruding upon the menopause and must be set aside.

Habits that revolve around sleep and hygiene, nicotine, alcohol and drugs, travel, hobbies and sports and more may have to be revised. Some even dropped. Pages 91–97 refer to these issues in greater detail.

Sex

From what you already understand about the hormonal, physical and emotional changes that are taking place at the menopause, it is clear that the sexual drives and gratifications are in for some sort of upheaval, or at least a regrouping. These new experiences and the physical changes that accompany them need not lead to sexual frustration and disharmony; they can actually lead to a more fulfilled and rewarding sexual life. More about that, too, in Chapter Seven.

Hormone Replacement Therapy

This is the centerpiece of MPX management. Most gynecologists now feel that hormone replacement therapy should be offered to every menopausal woman who has no insurmountable contraindication. The present methods of administration have been proven to be so safe and so effective that there is really little argument remaining against its regular use.

HRT has had a history filled with controversy. Both estrogen and progesterone equivalents were available for clinical use by the end of World War II. Progesterone was perceived to be of no value in managing the menopause since it offered no relief for any recognized menopausal problem. Estrogen, on the other hand, provided prompt and unmatched relief. Indeed, flushes and sweats, along with a variety of emotional problems, completely vanished as estrogen levels rose. (At that time, these urgent symptoms were the major recognized menopausal assaults, and the ones that needed to be treated.)

Accordingly, estrogen therapy for the menopause became very much in vogue. The hormone was widely given—often in unusually large doses—and for a while, women found relief from the unpleasant symptoms of the menopause.

But before long, snags began to appear in the forever-estrogen fabric. Cases of excessive uterine bleeding and of intravascular clotting (thrombosis) were reported in the literature in increasing numbers. Most devastating of all, an increased harvest of uterine (specifically, endometrial) cancer became a clear component of unilateral, prolonged estrogen administration.

Thus, by 1970, estrogen treatment of the menopause had fallen by the wayside, a victim not only of abuse but of unacceptable consequences.

During the decade that followed, significant clinical research involving the use of progesterone to allay the chronic irritative aspects of unopposed estrogen yielded good news. It was demonstrated, to almost universal agreement, that an estrogen-progesterone combination not only represented a safe menopausal treatment, but also actually appeared to protect the patient from uterine cancer, breast cancer and, perhaps, certain other problems.

Thus, the modern hormone replacement therapy program was born. Modern HRT almost always includes various *combinations* of *estrogen* and *progesterone,* although there is still some difference of opinion about the addition of progesterone after a hysterectomy has been performed. Moreover, the male hormone testosterone is now being used in certain circumstances. And that brings up the subject of HRT risks and benefits.

HRT Risks

What are the risks of HRT?

- Estrogen has been blamed for certain liver function impairments that adversely affect blood pressure, may produce gall stones and increase the chances of intravascular clotting (thrombosis). In modern dosage ranges, the chances of these problems occurring are very remote. Since oral estrogens are metabolized in the liver, as in fact all estrogens are eventually, they must be used cautiously or not at all when severe liver disease is present.

- High dosages of estrogens can and do alter sugar metabolism adversely. However, this usually occurs with higher dosages (birth control pills, for example) than with dosages used in the menopause. In fact, HRT is generally not contraindicated for women with diabetes. No long-term studies of the effect of *combined* estrogen-progesterones on carbohydrate metabolism have yet been completed.

- There is a clear, unshakable and deadly relationship between smoking and the use of birth control pills—which are, after all, synthetic estrogens and progesterones in fairly large doses. This relationship is absolute at age thirty-five and beyond. Modern hormone replacement therapy is in a lower dosage range and less synthetic. Thus the smoking relationship may or may not exist here. But why tempt fate?

• Estrogen has a positive, beneficial effect on blood lipoproteins by increasing the levels of cardioprotective high-density lipoproteins (HDL) and thus reducing the risks of cardiovascular diseases. The necessary addition of progesterone to HRT has been accused of blunting this beneficial effect. Accumulating evidence, however, indicates that this is transitory and—in the long run—the combination of both hormones serves cardiovascular protection better than estrogen alone. For a detailed look at progesterone, turn to page 61.

• If you are still fertile, can you get pregnant on HRT? Yes, you can. You can also win the Publishers Clearing House sweepstakes. Your chances are about the same in either event. But pregnancy CAN occur, so you had better ask your physician about possible birth control techniques at this stage of your life. Certain birth control pills can function at this time (for nonsmokers) as both a source of HRT and birth control (see page 112–13). Pregnancy, of course, is an absolute contraindication to HRT.

• Certain disorders of the reproductive organs prevent or limit the use of HRT. And HRT may nourish these problems.

Fibroid uterine tumors (myomata), very common benign growths that appear singly or in clusters on and in the uterine muscle, appear to be nourished and to grow in the presence of estrogen. They must be watched carefully if HRT is to be administered.

Endometriosis is another common gynecological problem that is certainly dependent upon estrogen for survival.

In this condition, which may arise when a woman is in her thirties, blood-filled cysts begin to appear on and around the uterus, tubes and ovaries and produce significant pelvic pain as they grow. Under the microscope the cysts appear identical to the endometrium that is normally found lining the uterine cavity. Endometriosis must be destroyed before HRT may be considered.

Cancer of the endometrium very definitely contraindicates HRT. Although the vast majority of present-day literature supports the claim that modern HRT does not cause this highly curable cancer, nevertheless estrogen will certainly nourish such a growth. Thus it must be removed before HRT can be considered. More about that later.

Testosterone therapy may induce facial hair growth and deepening of the voice and must be closely monitored.

Now, to the good news.

HRT Benefits

What are the benefits of HRT?

- Control of menopausal symptoms.

- Control of osteoporosis.

- Delay of arteriosclerosis and the attendant heart disease.

- Protection of the sexual life.

- Long-term studies indicate that the risk of endometrial and breast cancer appears to be actually reduced among women on a combined (estrogen-progesterone) HRT program.

That is certainly enough to make it all worthwhile.

Principles of HRT Administration

When to Start

Although some gynecologists prefer to wait until the MPX is well established (perhaps a year after the menses cease) before starting HRT, logic does not support such a stand. Significant discomfort and irreparable system damage may take place during that time. And nothing is gained.

Accordingly, most of us begin HRT during the PeriMPX, particularly since new evidence indicates that loss of bone mass may begin well before the cessation of menses (see Chapter 9).

Certain studies must precede HRT:

- A complete gynecological examination, including a Pap smear.

- A screening mammogram that shows no evidence of suspicious breast changes.

- In some cases, laboratory blood analysis for blood lipids (cholesterols and triglycerides) may be indicated.

How HRT is Given

Estrogen may be given in five ways:

- *Oral Pills.* Both naturally occurring female hormones (estrone and estradiol) are available—with some modifications—as oral tablets. "Premarin" contains estrone, some estradiol and certain other estrogen-like compounds. It is available in five strengths. "Ogen" is prepared from pure crystalline estrone and is available in two strengths. These two tablets are the most regularly prescribed estrone and estrone-like hormones. Generic substitutes were removed from the market by the FDA because they did not fall within a reasonable potency of the original compounds.

"Estrace," which contains micronized estradiol, and "Estinyl," which contains estinyl estradiol, are two commonly prescribed forms of estradiol and estradiol-like tablets. Again, generics are not available.

As in all oral medications, side effects may be a problem. Headaches and digestive disturbances lead the list but there are others. Read your package insert. Sometimes oral preparations simply cannot be tolerated and, even more rarely, they seem to be totally ineffective. Much has been made of the fact that all oral hormones must first pass through the liver as a "bolus" and much is deactivated in the liver before getting any farther. This is true, but the manufacturers have allowed for this inactivation in the dosage levels supplied. Certain liver disorders do require some other form of administration to spare the liver extra work.

- *Transdermal Patches ("Estraderm").* This newest form of estrogen replacement has been widely accepted in America and elsewhere. Pure estradiol is suspended in alcohol within a patch reservoir and weeps across several complex membranes to be absorbed through the skin. The patches come in two dose ranges and, therefore, two patch sizes. Worn below the waist, these patches are changed twice weekly. Although the manufacturers recommend that the lower abdomen is the preferred location, many women are applying the patches to their flanks or buttocks, feeling that these locations are more out-of-the-way and less of a nuisance. Estradiol picked up in the circulation transdermally from the patch does not bolus the liver and this may be an advantage. The benefits of patch-derived estrogen appear equivalent to all other externally derived estrogens.

Here are some extra points about the patch:
- Read the package insert carefully.
- The commonest nonmedication side effect of patches is local skin irritation (which is apparently more common in warm, humid environments) and failure of the patch to stick well enough.
- Be sure that you change your application sites as recommended. Be sure that the new site is dry—some women use a hair dryer to assure skin dryness. Moreover, some women put the patch on a flank area so they can bump that area hard against a wall after applying the patch—to help it stick!
- Patches may come off while you are bathing or swimming—or, more likely, in a hot tub. You may reapply the patch if its time is not up. If you remember, you can remove the patch before submerging and reapply it later.
- When your doctor is giving you a patch prescription for the coming year, be sure he gives you enough for a full year. Twelve packets will only last you forty-eight weeks. A year is still fifty-two weeks.

- *Intramuscular Injections.* Both estradiol and estrone can be given by injection. They are dissolved either in water (for quick but short effect—a week or so) or in oily substances (for slow release over several weeks). Usually one cubic centimeter (1 cc)—there are 30 ccs in one ounce—contains a therapeutic hormone dose. The water injections may be given into either arm or buttock muscles but oil injections are usually given in the buttock muscles only. Injection programs are rarely used for long-term hormone replacement—for a number of reasons: They are expensive, are usually inconvenient and peaks and valleys in estrogen blood levels are inevitable no matter how carefully the injections are timed.

- *Subcutaneous Pellets.* Although the subcutaneous implants of hormones for birth control have become a very successful and long-lasting (five years) technique, pure estrogen pellets as part of an HRT program have not. Work continues in this area but there are many problems to be solved. At this writing estrogen pellets are not generally available.

- *Estrogen Creams.* For many years, estrogen creams have been available in this country to be used as vaginal inserts with the goal being to increase vaginal health, lubrication and resiliency in estrogen-deficiency states. It has worked very well in this regard and continues to have wide acceptance—as it should.

  In general, this valuable tool is very important to many women suffering from a dry, atrophic and painful vagina and it should not be denied them—even in circumstances where estrogen often appears contraindicated. There is more on this subject later in this chapter.

  But it has a few disadvantages. It is messy and sometimes allergies develop to the suspending creams that are used. Just as in the transdermal skin patches, some of this vaginal estrogen is absorbed—more if the vaginal skin is thin. Thus, systemic estrogen effects may occur (such as endometrial buildup and uterine bleeding) and need to be anticipated and dealt with.

  In other countries estrogen creams are available to apply on skin surfaces as a lotion. These, like the patch, supply all estrogen needs. They are not available in this country. Some women's facial creams used to contain estrogen—supposedly to enhance the health and strength (and, therefore, beauty) of their facial skin. Such creams may still be available but they contain very little estrogen as far as systemic absorption is concerned.

- *Progesterone.* This hormone is almost always administered as a "progestin," which, you remember, is a synthetic progesterone-like group of hormone compounds. Progestin is used because pure progesterone is difficult to stabilize for oral administration and injections are expensive and inconvenient. There is a finely suspended oral progesterone now available in some areas and this could prove to be a solution to the oral route. When the progesterone-deficiency theory of PMS was in full bloom, sublingual lozenge and vaginal suppositories of progesterone were available in many communities. They had to be compounded by local pharmacies and had a very short shelf life.

The commonest progestin is medroxyprogesterone and is sold as "Provera" or "Cycrin." Generics are available. Other progestins are available and newer, even more natural progestins will soon be marketed. Some are already in American birth control pills.

Progestins (and, indeed, progesterone) often produce side effects similar to PMS. For this reason their addition to HRT programs may require considerable adjustment to fix a tolerable dosage.

- *Testosterone.* When this male hormone is considered useful in HRT programs (see pages 125–28), it can be given in a number of ways.
  - Oral testosterone tablets or sublingual lozenges are both available. The lozenges avoid the liver and are absorbed directly into the circulation while a significant portion of the tablets is lost to liver metabolism. Again, the dose range is adjusted for this fact.
  - Testosterone is often combined with estrogen in a single pill ("Estratest" is an example) in a balanced ratio that tends to offset some of the unwanted side effects of this male hormone.
  - Injectable testosterone is almost unavailable under any circumstances at this time. This represents a great

change in availability and has been caused by the tremendous abuse of this hormone by youngsters wanting to body-build. Thus, injectable testosterone has joined narcotics as a controlled substance!

- Testosterone pellets have been available but may be lost to the same fate as the injectable form.

Testosterone is included in some HRT programs to increase sex drive and response. It has certain side effects that must be watched for. These include body hair growth, acne, edema, weight gain and voice changes. Generally, if hormonal balance is achieved, most of these problems can be avoided.

HRT Programs

HRT is called for in several circumstances. Listed below are the circumstances and what is called for in each.

Uterus and Ovaries in Place

The treatment program here, at this point in our scientific knowledge, causes the menstrual cycle and regular periods to continue for some time—until later in the postmenopausal life. This is not always welcome news, for some women hope to dispense with all unused tampons and pads. Techniques such as laser ablation (destruction) of the endometrium are under study now and eventually may allow HRT to be instituted without the continuation of menstruation, but for the time being, the menstrual cycle must continue regularly and normally. Thus the hormones must be taken in a cyclic manner much in the same way as birth control pills—to produce cyclic bleeding. Also, again we must be reasonably certain that there is no substantial pelvic disease, such as fibroids or endometriosis, that might be nourished by the estrogen replacement.

What are the methods of treatment in this case? There are four basic alternatives; they are described briefly below.

- Oral estrogen tablets are taken daily for twenty-one days. During the last ten to fourteen days, progestin tablets are added to the program. Menstruation usually follows a few days after the last medication, and a new hormone cycle is begun on the fifth day of the flow. The dosages given vary somewhat dependent upon the physician's preferences and upon the responses of the patient. As the menopausal years go by, the hormone dosages and the combinations change, so that in women in their late fifties menses become but a trickle and may completely disappear. More on that when we discuss the postmenopause.

- Patches are generally used in a constant, uninterrupted manner—that is, two patches a week without cessation. In this program, progestagens are added orally for seven to twelve days every fourth week. Menstruation is usually regulated in this manner, but menses are sometimes difficult to adjust with this relatively new approach. It is certainly worth the combined effort of patient and physician.

- Injectable hormones are usually given only if other HRT forms of treatment are, for one reason or another, unacceptable. Most often the hormones are suspended in oil so that they will be slowly absorbed, and thus need be given only twice in one cycle. The initial dose contains estrogen alone and is given on the fifth postmenstrual day. A second injection containing both estrogen and a progestagen is given ten to fourteen days later, depending upon the patient's menstrual response.

- Subcutaneous pellets are put in place as frequently as recurrent menopausal symptoms indicate—usually at four- to six-month intervals—and progestagens are given by mouth at four-week intervals and for 10 to 12 days. Menstrual cycle adjustment may be difficult.

Uterus Removed But Ovaries Remain

It may be several years after the uterus is removed (hysterectomy) before HRT therapy becomes necessary. It depends upon the woman's age at the time of surgery and upon the health of her ovaries. Thus, a woman who sustains a hysterectomy at thirty-five because of fibroids may not need to start HRT for ten years (see page 16).

HRT is thus begun when menopausal symptoms appear, or when the vaginal hormone smear and/or the blood FSH and estrogen indicate failing ovarian hormone production. In actual practice, the appearance of recognizable MPX symptoms (flushes and sweats, for instance) is all the evidence needed to establish a trial HRT program.

In the absence of the uterus there is no need to provide cyclic hormone replacement since there will be no bleeding. This is a great advantage.

There is no evidence that HRT has any effect, good or bad, upon the aging ovaries.

The plans, then, are as follows:

- Oral estrogen tablets are taken daily without any interruption or change in the dosage level.

- Transdermal estrogen continues unchanged, being replaced twice weekly.

- Injections continue to be given at 2-week intervals but often can be spaced somewhat further apart.

- Subcutaneous pellets—should they be available—are replaced as often as necessary, at present up to 6-month intervals. If improved pellets become available, follow whatever replacement schedule the new limits require.

The role of progestins or progesterone in HRT after the uterus has been removed is, at present, a much debated subject within the profession. You remember that we talked about the history of HRT earlier (please see page 53) and that the experts finally discovered that estrogen should not be given alone—if the uterus was still present. A great deal of abnormal bleeding and, often enough, endometrial cancer followed unilateral estrogen administration. It still does. Why?

Progesterone "receptors" in the endometrium function by blocking the unlimited growth potential of estrogen through endometrial estrogen "receptors." That's how it works. Thus, both hormones are necessary to produce equilibrium and safety in the endometrium.

Now, then, there are both estrogen and progesterone "receptors" present in the breasts, in bone, in the blood vessels, in the skin and, indeed, in other important internal organs (as always, we're talking about women only).

Is it reasonable to assume that the uterus is the ONLY organ where these two receptors work in harmony and to the general welfare of the organs where they reside?

Evidence is gradually accumulating that to satisfy both receptors produces a healthier body environment. Here are some examples:

In the Breasts

- The survival rate of women with premenopausal breast cancer is significantly greater if the initial surgery is performed in the luteal (progestational) phase of the menstrual cycle.

- In tissue culture most breast cancer cell growth is inhibited by progesterone.

- Large doses of progestins are part of breast cancer chemotherapy.

- Men undergoing surgical conversion procedures to become female—more or less—are often given estrogen to enhance breast growth. No progestins are given to balance the estrogen-breast effect. There is a significant incidence of breast cancer in these men. Since breast cancer is exceedingly rare in men, this suggestive evidence of dangerous outcomes from unilateral estrogen stimulation in the male breast is most striking.

- Tamoxifen (Nolvadex) is a widely used agent to suppress breast cancer. The drug has been shown to raise serum progesterone levels. Read more about Tamoxifen in Chapter Ten.

- Progestins, used widely in oral contraceptives, have reduced the necessary number of breast biopsies in this country by 25,000 EACH YEAR.

- Two long-term studies comparing breast cancer rates in women taking estrogen alone, taking the combination of estrogen/progesterone or taking no hormones reveal that those on the combination have had significantly fewer breast cancers than the other two groups.

That is a fairly long dissertation on the role of progesterone (and progestins) in protecting the breasts against the unilateral use of estrogen in HRT programs. Even more will be said about this role in the chapter on breast disease further on in this book. It is a very important subject and one upon which there is still considerable disagreement.

In the Bone

- Bone loss can be as much as 20 percent of the total bone mass in the first ten postmenopausal years! Calcium and exercise are important but only with estrogen can the bone loss be retarded. Estrogen works by inhibiting "osteoclasts"—bone-melting cells. So it SLOWS bone loss. But it cannot build new bone. Guess what? Progesterone can and does. It forces osteoblasts—the bone builders—back to work and so bone is remodeled. Thus the two hormones work here in harmony as well.

In the Blood Vessels

- Progesterone has been accused of blunting the beneficial role of estrogen in raising HDL—the "good" cholesterol. Evidence now shows clearly that, again, the two hormones working in concert produce a better blood vessel response than either one alone.

Well, much more evidence exists to establish the point that I am trying to make—but I am lucky if you have read this far. Sufficient it is to say that mounting evidence supports the use of progesterone or progestins in all HRT programs.

Que sera, sera. We will see.

Accordingly, I feel that progestagens should still be given along with the constant estrogen program and in the same dosage range used in all the regular HRT programs.

Uterus, Tubes and Ovaries Removed

If the surgery removing the uterus, tubes and ovaries (hysterectomy and bilateral salpingo-oophorectomy) was for a cancer of the endometrium, hormone therapy may be absolutely contraindicated. (See below for further information.) If the surgery was for cancer of the cervix, HRT is not contraindicated. If the surgery was undertaken for the treatment of cancer of the ovaries, HRT must be decided upon on an individual basis.

Some gynecologists feel that HRT should not be used after this type of surgery if it was undertaken to remove extensive (or even early) endometriosis. That position, however, is not universally held, and many gynecologists begin hormone replacement therapy at once, in a modified way, usually employing large doses of progestagens or combining estrogen with the testosterone for the first few months. These programs must be tailored individually.

If there are no substantial contraindications to HRT, it should be started *immediately* after such surgery. The *younger* the patient, the *more important* this is.

The administration of HRT following this surgery is similar to that after an uncomplicated hysterectomy.

After Cancer of the Endometrium or of the Breasts

It has always been considered incorrect to give HRT to a woman who has sustained a cancer of the endometrium or the breasts. After all, both tissues are estrogen targets in the first place, and estrogen, when given alone, has been found to cause cancer of the endometrium where none existed before. Furthermore, as many of you may know, most breast cancers are tested nowadays after removal for hormone dependency and many are estrogen-dependent or estrogen targets, just like healthy breast tissue. For these and other reasons, leading experts have termed HRT ill-advised in such cancer cases, regardless of the severity of existing menopausal problems.

Recently, however, studies have begun to appear in which HRT has, in fact, been initiated in some women who have suffered these malignancies, provided

- At least five years have elapsed in which they have been free of any evidence of recurrence.

- Significant menopausal problems exist (osteoporosis, vaginal atrophy in young women, etc.)

- The patient requests it and is absolutely and completely informed of the known risks.

Although these programs are young and no hard and fast conclusions can as yet be drawn, HRT may become acceptable in such cases in the next few years. In this regard, there is recent evidence that proper HRT is safe to administer immediately after surgery for early (Stage I) cancer of the endometrium.

How Long Should HRT Last?

When, if ever, should hormone replacement cease? That depends to a large extent, upon which gynecologist you ask. This holds true whether the gynecologist is male or female. Remember, some don't think it is necessary at all, and some think it is only necessary for the first few years of the menopause, when bone loss is supposedly greatest and when symptoms are the worst. Finally, some believe you should take it as long as you live.

So we must go back to some of the basics. Your "menopause" only lasts a little while. The events that follow, however, last a long, long time. And so both of these things must be dealt with for a long, long time.

We have seen that the menopause represents an acute phase of ovarian decline and includes the cessation of monthly periods along with all the other symptoms—flushes, insomnia, fatigue, etc.—that surround it. Thereafter, there exists a hormone deficiency syndrome that induces or accelerates arteriosclerosis, osteoporosis, atrophic skin changes and multiple sexual dysfunctions in variable degrees. These are the postmenopausal years

(PMPX). This is where you are going to spend the rest of your life, and most women find that HRT makes it all more enjoyable and much, much safer.

The Cost of HRT

Hormone costs vary from one part of the United States to another and in different parts of any one community. And if generics are substituted, the prices may be even more unpredictable.

Here are some sample prices of hormones as posted in a local chain drugstore and as quoted by the Southwest area AARP pharmacy.

HORMONE	DRUG EMPORIUM	AARP
Premarin 1.25 mg	$11.85 per 30	$11.90
Estinyl 0.05 mg	$10.05 per 30	$13.45
Estraderm patch (0.1 mg)	$16.15 per 8	$18.60
Provera 10 mg	$18.15 per 30	$18.15
Estratest	$21.85 per 30	$19.30
Estratest ½ strength	$18.05 per 30	$15.95
Delestrogen Injectable (20 mg per cc)	$40.85 per 5 cc	$39.70
Generic injectable of Delestrogen	$8.75 per 5 cc	N.A.

Prices are lower when bought in larger quantities. Generic Provera is available and costs considerably less.

℮ Pause and Reflect

Gregory Goodwin Pincus is properly credited with the research that led to modern birth control pills. At about the same time he was doing this research he was also working with another group of substances that displayed strong *antihormone* properties. Dr. Pincus's unexpected early death led to a long suspension of any further study in this area. Recently, a new group of investigators has developed a marketable drug based on Dr. Pincus's original research with antihormones. Called RU-486, the drug can *obliterate* progesterone activity. It thus can serve as a birth control pill, but more importantly, it is so powerful as a progesterone inhibitor that it can regularly produce abortions in early pregnancy—up to the seventh week.

It is widely used for this purpose in other countries and is now being studied in the United States as an investigational drug under FDA guidelines. Whether or not it will ever be released here for any general use is a highly controversial subject. (These lines were written over four years ago and although a great deal more far-reaching research has been done, nothing has changed concerning this drug's use in America.)

——————————

When testosterone is given to female canaries, it will, in about 10 days, make them sing—giving them a capability that has always been limited to male canaries.

——————————

As patents for drugs expire, consumers have been provided with more choices between brand-name (pioneer) medication and generic substitutions. As far as hormones are concerned, here are some points to consider about generics:

• Substitution laws vary from state to state. Some require substitution if the generic is cheaper, some do not. In certain states there are other laws that may affect your ability to buy generic drugs. Your pharmacist knows these regulations.

- Generic estrogen tablets have failed to meet these requirements and have been withdrawn from the market.

- Inert substances used as fillers in the generic drug may be different from those used in the pioneer drug, and may therefore cause different side effects.

- A recent study of almost 1 million prescriptions involving both pioneer and generic drugs (collected from thirty-nine states) revealed that the pharmacy *always* paid less for the generic drug; the consumer *generally* paid less for the generic than for the pioneer, but sometimes she paid *more*, and prices of generics varied widely from one pharmacy to another and a continued search was no guarantee of finding the lowest price.

It has been estimated that the routine use of hormone replacement therapy in American women would save $3.5 billion each year in medical costs. This figure was arrived at by using data developed in countries in which the regular use of HRT for the menopausal population is more widespread than it is here. The cost of regular physical examinations plus the cost of hormone therapy was subtracted from the health services provided for women with osteoporosis, arteriosclerotic heart disease and other attendant complications that develop because of hormone deficiency in the absence of hormone replacement therapy.

These data do not even attempt to address the suffering and disability that hormone-denied women suffer from their consequent medical disorders.

A recent survey of almost 1,000 menopausal-aged women—which included a significant number of female gynecologists—revealed that while 62 percent of the gynecologists were on HRT, only 27 percent of the remainder had accepted hormone replacement (*OB/GYN News*, 1991).

Many strange stories have surfaced about the wandering of patches—some of which, I am sure, are familiar to you. Patches have been found floating in pools, hot tubs, regular tubs, fountains and in assorted restrooms. They have appeared on dogs, cats and various other pets—which could include husbands and/or consorts of whatever assortment.

One reported incident bears repeating. A husband and wife shared a pleasant, active evening in bed with some unusual results. The wife was brought to a hospital emergency room during the night complaining of chest pain, shortness of breath, syncope, flushing and other systemic symptoms. She had cardiac studies and, on the basis of the results, was admitted to the hospital. The next morning when an aide was giving the lady a bed bath, she noticed a nitroglycerine patch on her patient's backside. The patch belonged to the patient's husband and had been inadvertently transferred during the evening's intimate encounter! Removal of the patch was followed by resolution of her symptoms.

For assistance in finding your closest menopausal clinic, write:

The North American Menopause Society
c/o The Department of Obstetrics and Gynecology
2074 Avington Road
Cleveland, OH 44106–9814

6

LIFESTYLE ADVICE FOR
THE MENOPAUSE

Although it is the keystone, hormone replacement therapy is only one stone supporting our menopausal and post-menopausal lives. There is a great deal more to consider, some of which we should have considered a long time ago. But, for one reason or another, we have not. Now may be our last meaningful chance to change our habits, so let's get to it. This chapter offers some lifestyle suggestions for the menopause years and all the years that follow.

Nutrition

Proper eating habits are crucial to your good health at any time but are nowhere more important than in the menopausal and postmenopausal years. Our annual $416 billion assault on what the good earth produces for our enjoyment and fulfillment provides you and me with two topics to digest:

- what's a reasonable diet

- weight, weight, weight

Here follow some basic observations:

- The average American diet today is far too rich in fats (40 percent or more) and sugars (23 percent) and contains twice our actual protein needs.

- Our diet is sorely deficient in fiber-rich complex carbohydrates, fruits and vegetables.

- One hundred years ago, Americans derived two-thirds of their dietary protein from low-fat starchy foods like potatoes, rice, bread, cereals, dried beans and peas, and the remaining third from meat, chicken, fish, cheese and eggs. Not so today.

- Women have been "waved off" carbohydrates (starch) because they have been taught that carbohydrates are fattening and not nourishing. Untrue! A plain baked potato for instance, is a nutritional bargain. For 100 calories you get protein, many nutrients and fiber. If you add butter, sour cream, cheese, bacon bits and so on, you get fat and calories and weight. And the potato, of course, gets the blame. And if you french-fry this same one hundred-calorie potato you have a 300-calorie megachip.

- Other great carbohydrates include rice, beans, peas and lentils. All of these are also underutilized sources of protein.

- Every plant food, however, is deficient in certain proteins and so must be combined with other plant foods in any given meal to be nutritionally complete. Generally, combining a legume (beans, peas—even peanuts) with any grain (wheat, rice, oats, etc.) makes a protein-adequate meal. Soybeans come the closest to being totally "protein-competent." Surprisingly, pizza (good, fresh-ingredient, home-made pizza) is an excellent combination of plant and other proteins and valuable nutrients!

• Dietary fiber, which we liberally omit from our menus, comes only from plants. There are two kinds of fibers: insoluble and soluble.

   Insoluble fibers, like bran, add intestinal bulk, prevent constipation and protect against colon cancer. There are three types of insoluble fibers.

   There are four types of soluble fibers. These fibers slow the absorption of food, help lower cholesterol levels, decrease hunger and stabilize blood sugar levels. Thus they make excellent diet foods. They are found in whole grain breads and cereals, beans, peas, fruits and vegetables.

• Clearly, a diet inclined toward plant protein can reduce dietary fat, our most serious nutritional threat. *Fat* yields nine calories per gram, *starch* yields only four. Even alcohol yields only seven.

• High-fat diets are linked to increased heart disease and increased cancer of the colon, breasts and endometrium.

• There are health and weight advantages to consuming several (six) small meals a day. Fasting all night and skipping breakfast produces an inefficient, unhappy person with many metabolic problems.

• The U.S. Recommended Daily Allowances (RDAs) for women vary substantially from those of men. Women need fewer calories and less of most other nutrients, vitamins and minerals—save for iron. Menstruating women are nearly all borderline iron-deficient and require modest iron supplementation. Calcium must also be added to the daily diet once a woman reaches her middle thirties.

• A menopausal woman of average build (120 pounds) and height (5'4") requires 1600–2400 calories daily. In the postmenopausal years (over age fifty) those needs decrease to 1400–2200 calories daily.

So where does that leave us? Do we eat tofu and bok choy for the rest of our lives? Let's see what the latest "experts" suggest.

As you are well aware, our daily requirements are built—by the experts—into a pyramid, with the largest recommended dietary components at the bottom and all others wedged into increasingly small compartments as the pyramid rises. And the pyramid is rising—rising to a point where it may challenge the Tower of Babel, both in height and in quarreling.

But here it is, day by day:

• At the base, 6–11 servings of pasta, breads, rice and cereals.

• The second level, 3–5 servings of vegetables and 2–4 servings of fruits.

• The third level, 2–3 servings of yogurt, milk or cheese and 2–3 servings of meat, poultry, fish, dried beans, eggs and nuts.

• The fourth (the sin level), minimal and occasional fats, oils and sweets.

Left unanswered by the pyramid are many questions, such as:

• What kinds of milk, cheese or yogurt?

• What kinds of fruits and vegetables?

- What meats, poultry and fish?

- How big are the portions of all this stuff?

- Are canned or frozen fruits and vegetables as good as their fresh equivalent?

- Is there time and hope for a life after figuring these dietary things out each day?

Yes, there is some hope—but not much. Here are some more guidelines that may ease the burden a bit:

- Breads should be whole grain; cereals—unsweetened brans, oats, wheat, grits, cooked cereals; any rice or pasta.

- Fruits and vegetables: fresh, frozen or canned (in water) are mainly interchangeable; however, fresh is better.

- Milk is an undesirable adult food. But, if you must, drink skim milk. Even skim milk contains lactose, which adults can't digest without a lot of gas and cramps. Good yogurt doesn't have lactose, does have beneficial acidophilus bacteria and has more calcium and less fat than milk. Read labels.

- Meats should be the leanest available, poultry should be skinned. Try to concentrate on fish that are high in omega-3 oil—it is cardioprotective and found in cold water fish—halibut, salmon, snapper, trout and tuna. Don't fry meat, poultry or fish.

And here are even more tidbits:

- See lipids (page 82) for a full look at fats. But here let me say that less than 30 percent (20 percent is better) of your diet should be fat—and most of that should be unsaturated. So, if your daily calories allotment is 2000, no more than 600 of those calories should be fat. One gram of fat yields 9 calories, so your daily fat intake should be no more than 600 divided by 9—about 66 grams. Max. Read labels.

- Limit the use of nonfood fats such as margarine, butter, cooking oils, salad dressings and creams.

- Beware of labels such as "lite" or "cholesterol free." Some bakeries make their bread "lite" simply by slicing it thinner! Some foods advertised as "cholesterol-free" truly have no cholesterol but do have plenty of dangerous saturated fat in their formula. Read labels.

- At least half of your daily calories should come from carbohydrates. Select complex carbohydrates such as beans, peas, pasta, rice and vegetables. Your body has to work (burn calories) to digest them. Avoid "empty" carbohydrates such as white breads, cakes, sugar, etc.

- Eat a variety of fiber-rich foods: fresh fruits with their skins (where possible), vegetables and whole grains such as brown rice, oat and wheat bran.

- Increase your fiber intake gradually. Take one-half the recommended dose for a week. If you do not develop significant cramps or bloating, move up to the standard dose during the next week. Dietary fiber is very important in avoiding constipation, protecting you against colon cancer and helping to lower cholesterol. However, too much and too much too soon can alter your intestinal bacterial flora to your disadvantage and limit the absorption of your estrogen. More is not always better.

- Include 3–4 servings each day of calcium-rich foods: skim milk (if you must), low-fat yogurt, broccoli, sardines, canned salmon (with bones), greens. See page 151 for more calcium-rich foods.

• Limit your intake of sodium and sodium-containing foods.

• Avoid foods containing monosodium glutamate (MSG), sodium bicarbonate, sodium citrate and other sodium sources. Read labels.

• Use vitamin and mineral supplements with care and consultation. More is certainly not always better and most preparations are developed on the premise that you eat nothing of any value—ever. Avoid iron once you forever stop menstruation—unless you have a specific proven need for iron. Calcium will come from other sources (see osteoporosis). There appears to be real help from vitamin C and E as well as from beta-carotene in diminishing certain cardiac and malignant conditions. You may see these vitamins gathered into one pill and called "antioxidants." They are safe vitamin supplements. Some supplements—vitamin A and D, for instance—can be dangerous when overdone.

• If you drink alcohol at all, limit your consumption to one or two cocktails each day. Better still, have instead two or three glasses of red wine daily. Wine glasses (six ounces) of red wine, that is. And something (some fat, for instance) must be removed from your diet to make way for the added wine calories. There is pretty firm evidence that some of the ingredients of red wine (and it's not the alcohol) are cardioprotective. This evidence comes from several sources but became hot news when the results of a recent French study confirmed the fact. Their eating and drinking habits should have wiped out the French long ago with cardiovascular disorders—but such is not the case. It appears that red wine is the liquid guardian of their hearts. But—remember—there are a lot of other variables in French lifestyles so that red wine may be just one protective factor. Two-hour lunches may also make a difference! Remember, also, that more French people die of liver cirrhosis than does any other society. We'll talk about wine again in the chapter on aging. Meanwhile—*bon appétit!*

Those are the basics. You may want to consult *The American Heart Association Cookbook* and *Jane Brody's Nutrition Book* for further information.

Lipids

The amount of lipids (fats) now circulating in the blood of most Americans has become a major source of worry to you and me, to the medical profession, the Food and Drug Administration, the National Institutes of Health, the American Heart Association, the food (and beverage) industry and, most importantly, to the news gatherers. And *it is important*. So let's expand upon it just a bit.

- Cholesterol is the commonest and most worrisome blood fat. It is manufactured in our livers and is ingested in certain fatty foods. It is carried in the blood by lipoproteins— both in high-density (HDL) and low-density (LDL) forms. It is a very important and necessary substance. Without it, for instance, no hormones could be built within our bodies. No matter—the blood level should always be below 200 mg per 100 ccs of blood.

- HDL—which should be at a level of 65 mg or higher—is considered the "protective" lipoprotein. The higher the HDL proportion of your total cholesterol level, the less likely you are to have cardiovascular problems. The remaining cholesterol—LDL—is considered the culprit in

heart disease—the one that shingles your arteries with calcium plaques—and, in general, the lower its level in the
blood, the better (120 mg or lower).

- A total blood cholesterol over 220 is considered a red flag,
  over 240 a significant worry and over 260 a time for strenuous intervention.

- Triglyceride, another commonly measured and reported
  blood lipid, is very complex and often elevated in heavy
  drinkers, in people with gout and with certain inherited
  states. These lipids are apparently not as important in ar-
  teriosclerotic cardiovascular disease. Their level in the
  blood should be below 140 mg.

Now then, our cholesterol levels are out of hand because on
average too much of our diet—40 percent of our caloric intake—consists of fat and cholesterol. Here are some pointers:

- There are three kinds of fat—saturated, monounsaturated
  and polyunsaturated.

- Saturated fat is the most dangerous to our health and most
  effective in raising our blood cholesterol. It is found in animal foodstuffs (butter, cream, whole milk, eggs, cheese,
  beef, pork, poultry skin) and in two plant oils (palm and
  coconut) that are hidden in many of the prepared foods we
  eat and cook with. Foods listed as "cholesterol free" may
  indeed contain a significant amount of these unhealthy
  plant oils. Read labels.

- Monounsaturated fats such as olive, canola and peanut oil
  are much safer fats. Incidentally, some peanut butter is advertised as "cholesterol free"—which is true. There never
  was any cholesterol in peanuts!

- Polyunsaturated fats such as safflower, sunflower, corn and soybean oil are also safe fats. Some of these safe oils are often "hydrogenated" to make them solid so that they can be used in margarines and shortenings. This process makes the fats more saturated but still safe. Fish are an excellent source of polyunsaturated fats—particularly coldwater fish (salmon and tuna, for example) that are high in "omega-3 oil," which is felt to be cardioprotective. However pills containing pure omega-3 oil have not been found to be of value.

- Dietary cholesterol is found only in foods of animal origin and should be strictly limited.

- You should shoot for a diet containing less than 30 percent fat and try to approach 20 percent. Of that fat, no more than 10 percent should be saturated fat and/or cholesterol. Recent studies reveal that there are no significant metabolic differences between mono- and polyunsaturated fats. They both appear reasonably safe in your dietary fat compartment. Earlier in this segment we went over a simple way of figuring the total amount of fat in your daily diet.

- Your total daily pure cholesterol intake should be no more than 100 mg. Read labels.

- Your doctor has access to many medications that help to reduce blood cholesterol levels when all else fails or if the levels are dangerously high. These medications are expensive, often have serious side effects and should be administered with care and with your informed consent. Almost all elevated cholesterol levels will return to safety with proper diet, exercise and weight control and without medication.

There you have a lipid discussion in a peanut shell. It is a very involved topic and we have just scratched the surface. There are many excellent nutrition and cookbooks that will help you prepare great meals with a wide variety of tasty foods, supplying you with all you need to satisfy your taste buds, your stomach and your spirits—all without having to test the fat ceiling. I will list some of these books at the end of this chapter.

Overweight and Overage—Food in the Menopause

"And the weak shall inherit the girth."

That little homily is not necessarily true as I will try to point out to you. Nevertheless, excess weight gain and the menopausal years seem to have struck up a dependent and cozy relationship with each other. "I don't eat any more than I ever did—in fact, I eat less—but my weight keeps going up!" This is a lament heard thousands of times each day in physicians' offices. And it is a valid and painful lament.

The truth is that in the very late thirties or early forties, our metabolic rate begins to decline and so we burn less fuel to keep going. Food is our fuel and we need less and less food all the time—at least until age sixty-five or so when the drop finally levels off. Vigorous, sustained, regular exercise will raise our metabolic rate some and is just one more good reason to be physically active. Strenuous dieting, on the other hand, lowers our metabolic rate and therefore our need for fuel (food) and so actually makes it harder to keep off weight.

This is not a fun time for gourmets!

Here are some more metabolic and physiological facts that may grasp your attention:

- Fat tissue plays many important roles in our bodies. It insulates and helps to control our body temperature. It contributes to hormone production and storage (we already have seen that too much fat can contribute to estrogen excess and thus to serious problems) and, finally, fat cells store fuel. Now, the amount of fuel energy stored in our bodies as carbohydrates is about 300 calories—not enough to sustain us from one meal to the next. However, the fuel stored in fat—in just an average body—is about 100,000 calories. An obese person has enough fuel stored in fat to survive several months!

• The 35 Rule: it takes 3500 calories to produce a pound of fat. On the other hand, to lose a pound of fat by exercise alone requires that we run—rapidly—35 miles.

• There are two distinct fat patterns: "android" or male-like, where the fat is deposited in the central abdominal area (apple shape), and "gynecoid" or female-like, where the fat is predominantly in hips and upper legs (pear shape). Gynecoid fat is harder to lose but—for reasons as yet unknown—it is a safer fat, providing somewhat less risk for cardiovascular and diabetic disorders.

• No matter what fat pattern exists, obesity is associated with a much greater risk of illness and early mortality. Hypertension, cardiovascular disease and diabetes all flourish in a fat environment.

• Obesity is not simply due to overeating. Genetic, environmental, neurological and psychological factors all play a role. It is, however, intimately associated with our civilization and lifestyles. Couch potato has a double meaning.

Here are some other interesting facts about weight problems:

• At any given time, half of our menopausal population claims to be on a diet and about the same number are truly overweight. Evidence shows that the vast majority of us fudge (a bad word?) on our diets.

• We apparently eat less than previous generations but we don't move around as much. Heavy people don't use as much energy moving about as do their lighter counterparts. Aerobic exercise will achieve better weight loss results than either starvation or drugs.

• Some low-calorie diets offer as little as 900 calories daily. A diet below 1200 calories is almost never nutritionally adequate. Those of us on very low calorie diets should be under *adequate* medical supervision. Adequate medical supervision means being under the care of a physician who has special recognized training for, and interest in, weight-control programs.

  Low-calorie diets rarely achieve permanent weight loss. Yo-yo weight loss and gain is very dangerous.

• Some of us will gain weight on a 1200-calorie diet, some will lose. One contributor to this fact is the variable number and type of fat cells present in our individual bodies. The more empty fat cells present, the easier to gain and the harder to lose. Moreover, some types of fat cells release their energy more sparingly. And so it goes—or doesn't go.

In sum, it appears that obesity is not only the first disease of modern lifestyles, it is also a very common and serious disorder. Finally, most fad diets—as well as drugs—are dangerous and useless.

What to do? What to do?

Follow these simple guidelines and the menopause will go along more smoothly, more joyfully and less heavily.

- Find a calorie level that you can live with and that will stop further weight gain. Remember—if your total calorie intake per day is less than 1200, it is not nutritionally complete and supplemental vitamins and minerals are likely to be necessary. And at that level, you need professional help.

- Always break your fast with breakfast. Fresh fruit and grains/cereals are what you need.

- Have smaller, more frequent meals.

- Don't cheat on yourself.

- Concentrate on complex carbohydrates.

- Avoid empty calories—sugar, soda pop or too much alcohol, for instance.

- Avoid fad diets and appetite suppressants.

- Drink plenty of water.

- Don't cheat on yourself.

- Exercise, exercise, exercise. Besides everything else good that exercise does, it helps keep weight OFF.

The only permanent solution you and I have to healthy weight control is a properly designed and faithfully followed lifetime eating and exercise plan.

Your Personal Exercise Program

The physical activities required in daily life have vastly decreased in this century.

Machines, appliances, conveyances and conveniences have decreased our level of activity to the point where we now must manufacture, invent and prescribe things to do with our bodies in order to stay fit.

And here are some facts about exercise:

- Regular exercise, you remember, increases your basal metabolic rate by increasing your muscle mass. (Basal metabolic rate is the rate at which your body uses energy when it is at rest.) This makes it easier to keep your weight down.

- Osteoporosis can be retarded by regular exercise.

- Fitness and muscle strength increase resistance to disease (high blood pressure, diabetes, obesity, coronary artery disease), facilitate weight control and reduce tension.

- While it is true that physical activity will burn calories and help with weight control, remember that a brisk one-mile walk will expend only 100 calories, and that you must burn *3500* calories before you lose *one* pound of flesh!

Certain risks are involved in an exercise program, even a reasonable exercise program. Be aware of the following:

- Undiagnosed cardiac problems can lead to severe acute heart disorders with strenuous exercise.

- Severe—and permanent—muscle and joint injury and disease can result from the high-impact activity that is common to jogging and certain aerobic dance routines.

- Increased body core heat (hyperthermia) and excess water loss (dehydration) often follow inappropriate warm-up and cool-down programs.

Yet regular, proper exercise promotes general fitness, and involves three basic components.

1. *Aerobic endurance.* Any activity that forces the body to use more oxygen and increase the heart rate to 65 to 90 percent of maximal activity and that is engaged in for at least 20 minutes three times weekly will increase aerobic endurance. Fast walking ("wagging"), bicycling, swimming and low-impact aerobic dancing are popular ways of achieving this goal.

2. *Muscular strength.* This keeps you walking tall, protects your bony frame and increases your metabolic rate.

3. *Joint flexibility.* This also keeps you walking tall, but in addition helps you touch your toes and scratch your back.

These three physical goals cannot be met by any one form of physical activity. So you should involve yourself in a mix of exercise activity, including walking or "wagging," muscle resistance training, swimming, water exercises, bicycling, trampoline exercises and yoga.

These physical activities must be started slowly and followed regularly. There are many programs marketed in the United States directed toward women and their exercise needs. Many of them are dangerous and some are ineffective. The single best and safest program is on a videotape marketed (at cost) by the American College of Obstetricians and Gynecologists. Called "Balanced Fitness Workout," it can be purchased by writing:

The American College of Obstetricians and Gynecologists
600 Maryland Ave. SW, Suite 300 East
Washington, DC 20024-2258

Whatever program you settle upon should be measurably progressive and sufficiently enjoyable so that it becomes an acceptable and permanent part of your lifestyle.

No matter what degree of boredom may set into your exercise program, it will still beat a wash-tub, scrub-board, hand-wringer, clothesline and stove iron.

Habits

Most personal and intellectual habits are formed in the twenties and thirties. We are long past our twenties and even our thirties, and so all our habits—good, bad or indifferent—are rather firmly etched and entrenched. In fact they are as much a part of us, and as difficult to erase, as the lines on our faces.

Sadly, many of our habits are destructive of our health and greatly shorten our lives and life's pleasures. We have already talked about obesity. Now, in order to continue through the menopausal successfully, we need to address some other destructive habits.

Tobacco

Despite all you know, 35 percent of all women continue to smoke. Assuming that you don't chew tobacco, here are some points about tobacco worth remembering:

- Smoking is our nation's number-one health problem. *Nothing* else comes close.

- Secondary (sidestream, passive, someone else's) smoke is as dangerous as your own.

- Nicotine is addictive. Like cocaine, it creates dependence and compulsive use. Nicotine use is the most widespread example of drug dependence in our country. More women now are smoking than men, so more women than men are now dying of lung cancer.

- Smoking vastly complicates hormone replacement therapy, and many gynecologists cannot recommend HRT when their patient smokes. It is well known that smokers over thirty-five who take birth control pills increase their risk of stroke and heart attacks by an *astronomical* figure. Many of us feel the same is true when women combine smoking and HRT.

- Although physicians are giving up smoking at a remarkable rate, they are *dismally* failing their patients when it comes to delivering antismoking advice. Less than half of today's doctors are counseling their patients to quit.

What should you do if you smoke? You should give up smoking at once. But how can you give it up? There are two ways to quit smoking. First, make an internal resolution to quit. Nothing else is needed. Nothing else will work. Success rate? Ninety percent.

If the first step doesn't work, enroll in one of the many stop-smoking programs available in most every community. Some are free, some are expensive. About 20 percent of attendees quit smoking in the long run.

You may feel lousy for six to eight months. But you will never regret it.

Alcohol

Former First Lady Betty Ford has stated that "alcoholism is an equal opportunity disease." And she is so right. In fact, alcoholism is now increasing at a much faster rate for women than it is for men. Many, many reasons are given for this recent phenomenon, but social and general living problems, along with lack of self-esteem, seem to head everyone's list. As in everything else, both heredity and environment play significant roles in the development of alcoholism.

The highest proportion of heavy female drinkers is found in

the PeriMPX and the MPX group. Married women have the lowest overall rate and common-law wives the highest. Most married women over fifty with alcohol problems have no children at home and do not work.

If you are burdened with unmanageable alcoholic drives, great help is available from many quarters. Alcoholics Anonymous (AA) and Women for Sobriety are two magnificent self-help groups, and many professional counselors are also available in most communities.

What about those in the menopause years who feel that they can control their relationship with alcohol? Here are some points to remember:

- If you feel *anything* about your alcohol control at all, then it is probably a problem. You can never let down your guard with alcohol. Never.

- The menopausal years are times of particular stress when alcohol dependency can slyly take over in a very unobtrusive way. Be aware of how much you drink.

- Alcohol represents empty calories that immediately join your fat system. On the way there, the alcohol tears up a few liver cells, mugs the pancreas and shakes loose some brain cells—cells that sadly are gone forever.

- One or two drinks before your evening meal are *no* problem provided that

One or two drinks before your evening meal are *no* problem.

One or two drinks means *exactly* that. One or two. (The amount of alcohol in one or two drinks should total no more than that found in two ounces of 80-proof liquor. In addition, don't mix your drink with anything but club soda or water. All other mixers contain empty, useless calories.)

None of this evening escapade was preceded by daytime trips to the bar.

You are not overweight, have no other serious health problems that may relate to alcohol consumption and your one or two drinks are an adjunct to a healthy, well-balanced meal.

Here is my formula for an enjoyable integration of alcohol into your lifestyle:

- You must feel that moderate alcohol intake is an integral part of the enjoyment of good living. Particularly so with good wines, which are not necessarily expensive.

- If you are in reasonably good health, you could enjoy five ounces of wine with your lunch or dinner.

- Before dinner you might have one cocktail or highball. Don't mix with anything except water or club soda. Again, everything else that mixes contains empty and useless calories. At dinner, share a half carafe of an agreeable wine with an agreeable companion.

- Now that is the maximum. Nothing in the morning, no beer during the afternoon and nothing (nothing alcoholic) to get you off to bed. Anything less than the above suggestions is fine. Anything more is courting disaster.

- The moderate consumption of alcohol clearly has certain health benefits. The judicious use of alcohol provides us with a moderate tranquilizer and a reasonable mood elevator. It can reduce blood pressure and dilate blood vessels, thus improving peripheral circulation. We have already talked about the French study (and others) that demonstrate wine's cardioprotective role.

Moreover, I must add, from my personal experience, there are very few lasting visceral pleasures this life has to offer that exceed that of the moderate drinking of fine wine with treasured company in an appropriate setting.

Travel

As the nest empties out, more discretionary time and money may now appear on your horizon—so this may be a good time to broaden it. Today's travel opportunities are immense and this is probably the best time in your life to take advantage of them. With a few caveats.

- Be wary of sudden altitude changes. The most obvious is flying to a ski area from a much lower altitude. You are now more susceptible to altitude disorders such as mountain fever, and should spend at least one day getting used to your new environment before hitting the slopes. You will save on lift tickets and emergency room visits.

- When traveling abroad, find a good travel agent and stick to the beaten paths unless you are very adventurous, healthy and a regular foreign traveler.

- STDs (sexually transmitted diseases) abound in many foreign countries. For example, there are 250 million new cases of gonorrhea and 25 million new cases of syphilis worldwide each year. A recent report in the *Southern Medical Journal* entitled " 'Love Boat' Hepatitis," for example, reported severe episodes of hepatitis B occurring in wealthy, middle-aged women who had sexual liaisons with other passengers and crew members. As far as AIDS is concerned, it is epidemic in America and pandemic everywhere else. This incredible, modern-day plague is insidiously destroying whole cultures. The risks should keep us all from any dalliance or liaison—at home or abroad. So be particularly careful.

- Many other contagious and dangerous diseases lurk in foreign countries. There is a common misconception that immunization regulations set up by foreign countries are to protect the traveler. They are not. They are to protect the country. If foreign governments were interested in *your* health, they would publish their national disease statistics in their travel brochures. If you want the real scoop about the disease risks in foreign lands, contact the United States Public Health Service. Incidentally, allow yourself plenty of time for vaccines to become effective. Some take several weeks to reach adequate levels. Ask your doctor, the Public Health Service or the Centers for Disease Control in Atlanta (404–332–4559).

- I hope your food will have been harvested long *after* your wine but, just in case, be wary of wayside inns.

- If you plan to live in another country for an extended period of time you should ask the United States Public Health Service for its list of vaccines appropriate for that country.

- The International Association for Assistance to Travelers, 350 Fifth Avenue, New York, NY 10001, will, for a fee, provide you with a list of English-speaking physicians almost anywhere abroad.

- Remember how to manage jet lag: much water, little alcohol and light eating on board, and rest on arrival. Better to travel by ship.

- Take an extra, separate supply of your medications. When possible, leave all of them in their original bottles, clearly labeled with your name and the contents as written by your pharmacist. Some foreign customs agents take a dim view of unlabeled medications mixed together like jelly beans. Pack your original medications in your carry-on luggage and your backup supplies elsewhere.

- Incidentally, for the first time the Food and Drug Administration has approved a drug for the management of simple traveler's diarrhea. Bactrim (trimethoprim and sulfamethoxazole) is the drug. If you have no allergies to it, you might ask your physician to prescribe it for you to carry when you are traveling abroad.

All in all, have a nice trip.

Wellness and Fulfillment

This menopause book would not serve you properly without discussing the concept of total body wellness. The bedrock of good health is the integration of a well-managed body with a well-ordered spirit (psyche, soul—whatever you wish to call it). And, in the order of things, the spirit compartment is dominant. A strong and directed spiritual will to live and to control the flow and exuberance of bodily activity is the key to total wellness.

How is this spiritual goal achieved? Well, purposeful living requires us all to examine and consider the likely existence of a greater force in our lives and in the universal order than we can readily explain, a force that constantly provides us with a dependable and abiding haven (something we cannot provide for each other or that cannot be provided for us by creature comforts or visceral pleasures). Call this a spiritual force or whatever you will. Approach it by any rational religious or philosophical bridge you choose. If you accept it you are well on your way to a dominant spiritual life, without which there cannot be total wellness and with which all things are possible. And this includes an infinite source of unfailing power to help us control and conquer the destructive habits that chain us all.

This is valuable advice for the menopausal years and those that follow. Many of you already understand these things.

ℰ Pause and Reflect

Excess caffeine intake (caffeinism) produces a type of anxiety very common in women. Too often the cause goes unrecognized and improper treatment (tranquilizers, for instance) is prescribed. Gradual withdrawal from the culprit (coffee, tea, soft drinks and chocolate) is the proper treatment and essential to good health.

Caffeine is also linked directly to other health problems—some of them deadly. A recent study in the *New England Journal of Medicine* demonstrates a two- to threefold increase in heart attacks among adults drinking five or more cups of coffee daily.

——————

Always read labels! We've been through that catechism many times already. The United States government now requires that *all* prepared foods be labeled with nutritional information. Two types of information may be listed. Get out a milk carton or margarine tub and follow along.

- First, the "Nutrition Information per Serving" is listed. This shows the calories per serving as well as the protein, fats and carbohydrates present. The amount of cholesterol and of the various fats should also be listed.

- Second, the percentages of Recommended Daily Allowances (U.S. RDA) are listed. Some of these (iron, for instance) must be listed; others are arbitrary.

- The average American eats over one hundred times his or her daily sodium requirement.

- Women's fat deposits are harder to mobilize and reduce than that of men. This is because men have a higher level of a certain fat-mobilizing hormone. Wouldn't you know it!

- The amount of time that a child between six and eleven years of age spends before a television set is the most powerful predictor of his or her adolescent obesity. This year—for the first time—the U.S. government has recommended that children join adults in a low-cholesterol, low-fat diet. The problem is becoming that immense.

- Doctor Walter Willett at the Harvard School of Public Health is conducting intense research in an attempt to relate women's dietary habits to their health outcome—studies, by the way, that have long been women's due. Among his files are the toenail clippings of some 70,000 nurses! From proper analysis of these clippings (along with other supportive studies), Doctor Willett and his associates hope to learn more about the relationship of women's diet to many health problems, including breast cancer.

- Seafood is a good nutritional bet. The risk of getting ill from properly cooked seafood is about one in 2,500,000. However, the risk of illness when eating RAW seafood is much higher—one in 1,000.

• Monkeys fed a low-fat, low-cholesterol diet were 50 percent more likely than the regular-diet monkeys to grab, bite, shove and otherwise torment their buddies.

• The effect of alcohol upon sexual arousal of, and pleasure for, women has been the subject of jokes, locker-room discussions and sophmoric conjecture for ages. But a closely controlled study shows that women who thought they had consumed alcohol felt more aroused—whether they had actually consumed alcohol or not. Conversly, women who actually consumed alcohol had less and less arousal as they increased their consumption of liquor. The old adage "Candy is dandy but liquor is quicker" may be just that— old.

• Get this: The most addictive of ALL drugs is nicotine— followed in order by ice, crack, crystal meth, diazepam, alprazolam, methaqualone, secobarbital, alcohol, heroin, crank, cocaine, caffeine, PCP, marijuana and ecstasy. More Colombians are destroyed by nicotine than Americans by cocaine!

• For pleasant, healthful cooking sources:
  • *Jane Brody's Nutrition Book* (Bantam Books).
  • *The American Heart Association Cook Book* order from: 7320 Greenville, Dallas, TX 75231.
  • *Cooking Light Cookbook,* Oxmoor House, Inc., P.O. Box 2463, Birmingham, AL 35201.

7

THE MENOPAUSE AND
THE BEDROOM

Sleep

A good night's sleep during the menopause, as at all other times of your life, is very important. One of the first good-sleep principles is to be very careful what gets between the sheets with you at night. You must learn to empty your mind of the frustrations, fears and angers that the day has heaped upon you. Bring them in with you and they'll irritate you all night and still be there in the morning. Believe me, you *can* learn to put them out with the cat.

Certain things work against your chances of a good sleep at menopause time. By far the most common is, of course, night sweats. Night sweats are almost totally preventable by adequate hormone replacement therapy.

Here are some more sleep helpers:

- Use your bedroom for sleeping and loving only. Put your TV set elsewhere. No reading, writing, knitting or TV watching in bed.

- Go to bed when you are sleepy but try to get up at about the same time each morning. Even if you have slept poorly, try not to nap during the day.

- As I said, leave the thoughts, torments and events of the day behind, and fantasize. That can mean anything from counting sheep to counting the hairs on Casanova's chest. Boring fantasies (like the sheep) seem to work better for some individuals than do the exciting ones. Use any fantasy that gets you involved and that works for you.

- Avoid exercise (except sex), caffeine and alcohol after you finish your evening meal. Alcohol may relax you into falling asleep, but the sleep is usually not deep or lasting.

- Avoid dependency on sleeping preparations of any kind.

- "White noise" sometimes helps a poor sleeper drop off pleasantly. Such things as ceiling fans, tapes of rainstorms and safe-harbor and seashore sounds often have this effect. They also serve to block out unwanted background noise—like someone else's TV, cat, dog or snoring.

- Don't eat just before retiring or retire just after eating.

- If all else fails, visit a sleep clinic. Little Rock, which is a small city, has at least three sleep clinics, so these clinics are not uncommon. Most audiovisual stores rent sleep-training tapes, or can get them for you.

Sex and Loving

A great revolution has occurred in our sexual lives and attitudes since the days when a British mother's only advice for her betrothed daughter was "Close your eyes and think of England." The revolution has brought many changes—some bad, most good—in our sexual activities and customs. One of the best changes involves women's freedom to develop and experience their own uninhibited and unfettered sexual expression and pleasure. Now, as the menopausal and postmenopausal ranks swell, questions about continued sexuality become increasingly common.

Menopausal women can expect several sexual changes that normally occur as time goes by. For example, you may have an increase in sexual drive as estrogen levels drop and androgen (male-like) hormone levels persist. The ovaries do produce testosterone—about one tenth that of the male. An increase in sexual drive is not regularly noted, however, and many times the reverse is true. This is certainly the case if the ovaries are surgically removed or destroyed by disease. Under normal circumstances, sexual drives continue in women into the seventies and eighties, but at decreasing levels.

Sexuality and sexual drive are very complex issues and cannot be dismissed in a few paragraphs. Much is being written about estrogen and testosterone levels, societal attitudes, lifestyles, general health and other factors affecting our sexuality as we age, but for the most part it doesn't add to our knowledge—only to our confusion.

As an example, much study is now going on concerning the sexual effects produced by a simple hysterectomy, which conserves the ovaries. The consensus at the moment (and this very broad, very inclusive consensus was reported by a female gynecologist) is that the removal of the uterus with proper conservation of the ovaries should not result in an increase in psychosexual problems. Although that is the majority opinion, there is still wide disagreement in this sensitive area, and there is increasing evidence that the ovaries that remain behind after a hysterectomy will fail at a significantly earlier age. Finally, very little study has been given to the sexual effect that a hysterectomy may have upon a lady's consort. Some evidence does exist that, in certain cases, such surgery may color or alter a partner's sexual response thereafter. There appears to be an ethnic bias in this area. More study is on the way.

Testosterone is available for those women who suffer from a significant loss of sexual drive during and after a natural or surgical menopause. Proper dose levels of this male hormone—in combination with estrogen—will generally prevent excess hair growth and other masculinizing effects. Regular medical monitoring and dose adjustment are necessary.

Excitement and arousal, which are usually marked by vaginal lubrication and swelling, also change. Sexual arousal now often requires more foreplay and local stimulation; indeed, without HRT, natural lubrication may not be possible. In addition, if HRT is absent, vaginal skin atrophy occurs and leads to painful intercourse along with many other local discomforts. You've read about this already.

Orgasm continues but "time-to-orgasm" may be lengthened without HRT. Menopausal and PMPX women may continue to experience multiple orgasms as before.

Yet there are several other factors in your new sexual equation. First, what about him? If he is your partner of long standing and about your age, his sex drive started declining several years ago and will diminish more rapidly than yours. In addition, although about 80 percent of seventy- to eighty-year-old men claim sexual activity, arousal takes much longer, and usually involves some form of direct stimulation of the penis along with great care to achieve and maintain erection. These changes, mind you, are gradual in onset. Finally, the latent time between successful orgasms increases so that by age sixty, male orgasm cannot be repeated for about two days. This is sharply different from the female's experience. While testosterone medication will increase men's drive somewhat, it does not increase their erectile or orgasmic ability.

It is clear that many diseases that tend to congregate in and plague our senior years will have a significant effect upon sexual drives and sexual pleasure.

- Diabetes, heart problems, hypertension, obesity—these common disorders plus their complications plus medications used in their treatment—all these things may have a profound and adverse sexual effect. In both sexes. When these disorders are properly controlled, there is a much better chance of fulfilled sexual expression.

- Arthritis by limiting pain-free motion will not only curb the bearer's pleasure but, by fear of producing pain, may also curb her partner's responsiveness. Women who suffer from arthritis—particularly rheumatoid arthritis—may enjoy sexual congress in the morning, just after maximum mobility is achieved and before the ever-present fatigue sets in. Hot tubs and big Jacuzzi tubs are places where joints can be made to move with less discomfort. Sexual experimentation in these devices should be pursued unless forbidden by a physician or therapist. For specific help ask your doctor or call for a booklet called "Living and Loving," published by the Arthritis Foundation (1–800–283–7800, or call your local chapter).

- Several heart conditions tend to limit men's sexual responsiveness because of their fear that their cardiac condition may be severely aggravated by sexual excitement. More on that in a following section devoted to men alone!

I have already mentioned that many of the medications now being used to treat major health problems can have a dampening effect on sexual activity. These may include drugs that treat anxiety, depression, heart disease, hypertension and fluid retention. Sedatives also act as sexual inhibitors. HRT and testosterone are the only medications that will help support a continuing sexual life—although there is some evidence that one antidepressant (Bupropion) may have some aphrodisiac effect.

While on the subject of aphrodisiacs, many substances have been used since the beginning of time to enhance and increase sexual pleasure and preformance. Yohimbine is a prescription drug that is sometimes used to treat impotence and loss of libido. It is apparently safe and is sometimes effective. Most street drugs (except heroin and methadone) will initially enhance sexual pleasure but destroy it—and everything else—with prolonged use. Alcohol is a sexual depressant and is a serious and common cause of sexual dysfunction in both sexes.

Researchers are looking for an aphrodisiac that is safe and dependable so that they can treat the wide variety of sexual problems that exist today. See more about aphrodisiacs in Pause and Reflect at the end of this chapter.

The last, and perhaps most important, factor in your new sexual equation is the quality of your partnership. This is really the key to a rich—or barren—sexual life. All of the factors noted above, taken together, depend upon the depth and stability of the union along with an understanding of the changes that accompany aging. An unstable relationship filled with pent-up angers and frustrations will surely fly apart at this time. A healthy, mature, growing relationship will be able to explore more erotic and sensual sexual depths than ever before.

How Best to Approach Sexuality in the Menopause and Beyond

Remember what you just read, particularly two things: First, your same-age mate will likely be undergoing a decline in sexual drive more rapidly than you. Second, this is particularly true if you are being supported by HRT and he is not. At the present time, HRT (testosterone, in this case) is not generally recommended for men.

If both partners understand the age-related changes that normally take place at mid-life, they will be more likely to prevent serious sexual and marital problems down the line. Thus, as an example, if you both understand that it now takes direct stimulation of his genitals (orally, mechanically, thermally, digitally or whatever it takes) in order to produce an erection, then no one's feelings are hurt. *You* don't feel you have lost your appeal and *he* doesn't feel that sex, as he knew it, is over.

On the above basis, minor sexual problems can generally be worked out at home in bed. Major sexual problems that occur at this time are generally a result of serious disorders in your relationship and require professional sex and marriage counseling.

Vaginal penetration is neither the beginning nor the end of sexual lovemaking. It sometimes cannot be accomplished—at any age. Shared intimacy, sensual pleasure, holding and caressing are often equally meaningful and enjoyable.

Sex should not be performance-oriented, but rather pleasure-oriented. For both of you. Together you should seek an erotic arousal environment, comfortable to both, with no demands and only the exploration of new pleasures.

Special Situations

Some special situations may affect the ways in which you express your sexuality. For instance:

- May–December relationships require special attention. If your loved one is much older than you, it is necessary that you make generous allowances for his sexual limitations which, as you are aware, are real and progressive.

- If your spouse becomes permanently impotent because of medical or other reasons, and if it is the wish of both partners, penile implants are now a reasonable solution. However, without any help, many older men remain sexually active and erectile well into their eighties.

- Now, then, the reverse. A much younger husband, biologically, should be the ideal sexual companion for a mid-life woman. That is probably the case, although I do not have the statistics to prove it. What *is* proven, though, is that the nonsexual complications of this kind of relationship are difficult to maintain.

- Removal of the ovaries—or suppression of their hormone function—is considered to be a part of the treatment of both cancer of the breast or of the uterine lining (endometrium). Such treatment, therefore, induces an abrupt menopause with all its systemic and disabling effects. Among these effects is the onset of a dry, thin vaginal wall that will not accommodate sexual activity without significant and often intense discomfort. A few physicians, in an attempt to help their patients, will prescribe vaginal estrogen creams to relieve these symptoms, but most have feared the legal consequences of supplying estrogen in any form should the cancer recur for any reason.

Recently, however, this distressful situation has undergone some encouraging changes:

- Women blessed with a five-year arrest of breast cancer have been offered—and many have accepted—the institution or reinstitution of HRT. This is a very complex decision and should involve very informed consent and agreement on all sides that the disabilities caused by the absence of HRT (sexual, vascular, bone, etc.) are destroying the quality of life for this already burdened woman.

• HRT is being offered to women almost immediately following surgery for early cancer of the endometrium instead of withholding it for the usual five postsurgical years. Statistics are rapidly being accumulated revealing the safety and the many benefits of this program. This is truly a remarkable change.

Loners

Some women live alone by choice, but an increasing number find themselves alone as a result of being widowed, divorced or separated. In any case, sexuality and normal sexual drives remain a fact of life that must be dealt with. Women who live alone by choice have already met that problem one way or another. The newly divorced or widowed woman at mid-life has but few choices to resolve her new problem.

Masturbation is a safe, harmless way to release sexual energy and pressure. Any nonirritating lubricant and a vibrator are all that is needed. Masturbation is not immoral, unnatural or dangerous.

The Junk Male

There is a pack of predators skulking in the wings waiting to help newly divorced or widowed women to continue their sexual life. Members of this happy little brand of do-gooders not only carry with them the desire to help you obtain continued sexual relief, but may also carry with them every known sexually transmitted disease. Which is about the only thing you will get out of the relationship. Watch out for these men.

Forming meaningful new relationships has its own problems, too. Multiple relationships are dangerous, if for no other reason than health. Remember, a condom covers only the penis. The mouth and hands and everything else lie bare and can carry disease—and *do*.

Even forming a relationship that you wish to be continuing and monogamous can be dangerous insofar as sexually transmitted diseases are concerned. Any male interested in you has probably been interested in and active with other women. It is a difficult challenge to face. And I don't have the answer. Today, there probably is no answer.

Lesbians

Relationships between lesbian women are much more stable than those of male homosexuals. Since sexual aging and drive generally proceeds at the same rate in a lesbian relationship, there is much less likelihood of sexual disharmony than in a heterosexual relationship. Another interesting point: Lesbian women complain much less of menopausal symptoms than do their heterosexual counterparts.

Sexually Transmitted Diseases at Mid-Life

In today's sexual climate, concerns about STDs (sexually transmitted diseases) during and after the menopause years are understandable, particularly when we read that 10 percent of all female AIDS victims are over fifty!

Monogamous couples have no need to fear AIDS—unless

one of them injects IV drugs or does work that brings her (or him) into contact with blood or other body fluids from AIDS patients. People working in these environments are acutely aware of the hazards and protective responsibilities. AIDS contracted by blood transfusion is now extremely rare.

Non–drug-abusing monogamous couples need have no fear of contracting any sexually transmitted disease (STD) unless one of the partners is an asymptomatic carrier of an STD from a previous relationship. Of these STDs, condylomata (HPV, or genital warts) is the most prevalent, followed by the relatively harmless herpes virus. These two STDs are increasing rapidly, particularly the human papilloma virus (HPV, or condyloma). HPV is gradually taking over the world while AIDS hogs the spotlight. HPV may produce warts at the vaginal entrance or may—without any symptoms—take up residence in the cervix and vagina and there produce premalignant and malignant changes. Thus, HPV is causing a major epidemic of cancer of the cervix in youngsters (who are very sensitive to the virus and are more sexually active) and it has now made its way into the menopausal generation. Regular Pap smears are your major source of protection and their annual procurement—whether you have a cervix or not (remember, the vagina is often involved)—is very, very important, no matter what else you may have been told or who told you.

Of the bacterial STDs, chlamydia, gonorrhea and syphilis are all increasing in the MPX population, but at a slower rate than the virus infections. And they are generally easier to treat. The symptoms, signs and treatment of these STDs are far beyond the scope of this book. But any unusual discharges, ulcers, sores, growth, warts, redness or swellings in the vaginal and rectal areas need prompt medical attention.

Most times, when you ask a new partner about his sexual disease history, you will hear what he wants you to hear. Nothing else. And remember, safe sex is not just having your partner wear a condom, since it covers only his penis, which is but a tiny part of his sexual equipment. Safe sex is a long-standing monogamous relationship.

Birth Control

Although research has indicated that couples become infertile when the woman reaches about forty years of age, don't depend upon it. I have delivered many babies for women well into their forties.

What is true is that fertility in the forties is vastly diminished by reduced sexual activity, declining male sperm counts and irregular and infrequent ovulation.

Even though the likelihood of pregnancy is reduced, very few women at menopause have active reproductive goals, so concerns about birth control are very real.

Sterilization has become the birth control method of choice for both men and women during the past-thirty years as techniques have become safer, simpler and surer. Today, surgical sterilization is chosen by 35 percent of women and 25 percent of men. Tubal ligation in women fails only by 0.2 percent and vasectomy in men fails by only 0.1 percent.

Modern, low-dosage birth control pills are, for nonsmoking, otherwise healthy women, a reliable, safe, effective method of menopausal birth control. Why?

- They are very effective (failure rate: less than 3 percent).

- They are very safe. Scientists have been unable to demonstrate any link between the modern pill and any female cancer.

- In fact, modern pills protect women against uterine (endometrial) cancer and ovarian cancer, even for years after they stop using the pill. This is a totally unexpected and unplanned oral contraceptive bonus.

- Protection is also provided against ectopic pregnancy, pelvic infections, simple ovarian cysts and iron-deficiency anemia (less menstrual flow).

- 25,000 fewer breast biopsies are performed each year because birth control pills suppress simple breast cysts.

- Menstrual cramping virtually disappears.

- Birth control pills supply adequate hormone replacement for the early menopausal years.

The intrauterine contraceptive device (IUD) has been reintroduced to the American market recently. All IUDs were removed from the market some years ago because of alleged bad results with one of them. IUDs are very effective in the menopausal years (4 percent failure rate). IUDs have been accused of reducing fertility and increasing the risk of sexually transmitted bacterial diseases. Reduced fertility is not important at this time in life and the risk of STDs is a matter you must deal with personally. You have the necessary information.

In view of the decreased fertility that accompanies most menopausal states, barrier methods—although less effective—may suffice for you. Thus condoms (14 percent failure), diaphragms (18 percent), cervical caps (18 percent), sponges (18 percent), spermicides (20 percent) or withdrawal (forget it) may work for you.

Failure is variably dependent. The IUD, for instance, is virtually beyond the bearer's control. The others are a blend of user and technique failures and almost impossible to assign.

When to Quit?

When should you stop using birth control? The answer must come from your own gynecologist.

Generally speaking, oral contraceptives—as well as HRT—will make women continue to have regular cycles long after they are no longer fertile. Stop the hormones and the periods will stop. But, of course, you don't want to stop the hormones. Sooner or later, however, you will want to switch from OCs to regular HRT. HRT is a generally adequate, though not proven, contraceptive for women from the mid-forties on.

IUDs may safely be removed and barrier contraceptives safely pitched after one year of amenorrhea (no periods). Most are generally discontinued before that time.

Gentlemen's Quarters

> "Why can't a woman be like me?"
> —Professor Henry Higgins in *My Fair Lady*

Dear Women: The messages that follow in this section are directed to the men who love you and care for you. The intent of all that it contains is to help them understand the vital changes and difficult bridgeheads that beset your body and soul as you pass through the menopause and beyond. Understanding the whole process will—I sincerely hope—help them to support and ease you through the critical times when everything is flashing "TILT" before your eyes.

Please ask the man in your life to read this section. He can even write to me if he needs further information. But ask him to read it. Fold it in the sports section of your paper, put it in the bathroom, by his side of the bed, in his shirt drawer, in his workshop, his briefcase, his tackle box, in the wet bar, taped to the TV remote or his Grecian Formula bottle . . . anywhere that keeps it before him. Unlike Professor Higgins's wish above, your man surely doesn't wish you to be like him!

Gentlemen, it is time that we had a serious discussion about the wondrous women (created for us by our Maker from one of our lesser ribs) that fulfill our lives and give them meaning. This is a very difficult subject to discuss and you have already—at this very early point—accepted a dangerous misstatement. Regardless of what you may have thought, Rebecca Carr and her associates have established by genetic testing of DNA found in fossils that, in spite of Genesis and all that it says, the first truly *Homo sapiens* creature came from Central Africa about 200,000 years ago. And—get this, you men—it was a WOMAN! And one more thing you need to digest is that while women's brains are slightly smaller than those of men (because their bodies are slightly smaller), our ladies' brains have been decisively shown to function much better than ours—using either side!

Remembering these things, let's move on.

The Male Menopause

We need to try and set this subject to rest before moving on. Is there, indeed, a male menopause? And if there is, should it not, in all fairness, be called the womenopause? Forget that. Here's what I know:

- At the menopause, women's estrogen production ceases very abruptly and causes profound destructive changes as this book outlines. Men's production of testosterone, on the other hand, peaks in their early thirties and gradually declines as the years go by. There is no abrupt cutoff point.

- The slow decline in testosterone is accompanied by a slow decline in sexual drive and performance and by a slightly decreased risk for cardiovascular disease. Many other factors such as general health, habits, obesity, stress and so forth contribute heavily to both of the above situations.

• The administration of replacement testosterone to men in their middle years and beyond is just now being studied. In the past, the risk of prostate cancer and the risk of augmenting cardiovascular disease was considered to be too great for the institution of testosterone replacement therapy. Incidentally, testosterone has been abused by adolescent boys and by some older "sports" figures. Massive, eventually destructive doses are taken by them to increase muscle mass and body size. As a result of this dangerous abuse, testosterone is now a controlled substance—like morphine!

• In our middle years, we men often face multiple social, personal, medical, sexual and career goal conflicts that bring us—often abruptly—to a confrontation with our own mortal nature. This stress—added to the daily stress of our world—often produces some menopausal-like symptoms. Such symptoms may include depression, irritability, insomnia, anxiety and angst. Flushes and sweats, however, are most unlikely and, if they do occur, are generally related to some other health problem—high blood pressure, for instance.

Personally, I would hope that some hormone therapy could eventually become safe and accessible to men. In this ONE research area much more study has been given to women's needs.

Cycles

We are all bound up by cycles: circadian (thus jet lag and swing-shift lag), business, weather and astronomical cycles, as examples. In regard to the last one—astronomical—a cycle is considered one rotation of a heavenly body. One heavenly body is our moon and, for reasons known only to nature, women's lives are cyclically bound to those of our moon—28 days. Of course, there are variations of three or four days on either side, but, by and large, just about every 28 days one complete menstrual cycle takes place. This one cycle produces profound changes in women's physiology and function.

- There are intense changes in the secretion of the various female hormones—FSH and LH from the pituitary, and estrogen and progesterone from the ovaries.

- In mid-cycle an egg ruptures from one ovary.

- During a cycle the uterine lining grows to receive a fertilized egg. If there is none, menstruation occurs.

- A new cycle starts.

- Birth control pills will somewhat alter this hormone cycle but contain variations upon both estrogen and progesterone. They do not alter the length of each cycle but instead tend to make cycles more regular.

- At the menopause, these cycles and the hormones they produce abruptly disappear.

Two important conditions relate to our women's cyclic hormone life:

Premenstrual Syndrome (PMS) is a real affliction variously affecting well over half of all women. This is what it's about:

- Starting usually about 7–10 days before a period, symptoms occur such as breast tenderness, generalized swelling, depression, irritability, headaches, depression. All these things and many others mount as the menses approach, then melt away after it begins.

- There is no known single cause for this syndrome. Treatment, therefore, is symptomatic and not always satisfactory.

- Until research provides something better, we can help women by avoiding controversy, confrontation, attempts at mutual decision-making and social and family obligation—until after period time. Even when PMS seems to encourage us men to do the reverse.

The Menopause

- Estrogen depletion occurs abruptly when the ovaries fail at menopause and instantly if the ovaries are surgically removed—incidentally, many, many more women have ovaries removed than men have testicles surgically removed. Both are considered castration.

- Regardless of how it comes about, the menopause has profound and destructive effects on women's health.

  - Flushes and night sweats can severely hamper lifestyle and sleep time for many years. Also, significant emotional changes are not unusual. Such emotional changes are not related, as often suggested, to the "empty nest syndrome" nor to loneliness or lack of purpose.

  - Bone loss accelerates at a tremendous pace with absolutely no visible symptoms.

  - Hardening of the arteries also accelerates rapidly— again, without apparent symptoms for years.

  - Over time, the vagina becomes dry, vaginal infections common and sexual intercourse very painful. Psychosexual problems may also increase.

- Hormone replacement therapy (HRT) is very important for the vast majority of menopausal and postmenopausal women who have no contraindications for such therapy.

- Emotional support and understanding by those of us who love them is probably the most important care of all. We must support regular examinations, mammograms, bone studies and all the things that will help preserve the lifestyle and freedom of our beloved companions.

Mature Sexual Bonding

There are very few better, more fulfilling forms of interpersonal communication than loving sex. Everything should be done to preserve this communication by both partners in any mature, meaningful relationship. Age should not be considered a barrier to this consumation, although it may alter some of the basics.

- Sexual drive usually diminishes in both sexes—gradually in men, sometimes more abruptly in women. Both often notice a delay in orgasmic response.

- The male drop. Impotence is, to us men, a devastating problem. Uncommon before thirty-five (1 percent), it becomes more prevalent (20 percent) by the sixties and common (80 percent) by the nineties. In the beginning erectile failure may be intermittent but generally proceeds on to constant failure unless therapeutic intervention is sought. The causes of this condition are multiple—psychological, neurological, vascular, glandular, medications, social drugs, aging—or any combination of those factors. Impotence, from whatever cause or causes, may be reversed in many cases by proper medical care or increasingly successful surgical procedures. Meanwhile, you and your partner help one another by not being preformance-oriented toward each other and by experimenting with genital and general lovemaking techniques discussed earlier in this chapter. Hang in there.

• Most cardiac conditions—including previous heart attacks, bypass surgery, pacemakers and the like—should not interfere with a normal sex life. The stress of a sexual encounter (unless it is out of bounds) is no greater than walking up a flight of stairs. Ask your cardiologist for confirmation of this data.

• Remember: Without hormone replacement, your partner's vagina may become very dry, thin and strictured. Vaginal infections may become common and penetration in any manner may be very painful. Various special lubricants (Gyne-Moistrin and Replens, for example) are available but the best treatment is local and/or systemic HRT if there are no serious contraindications. Oral and manual stimulation should be very gentle. Go easy. And lovingly experiment. One important caution: Rectal sex should not be a part of your sexual play—unless you are in a long-standing, completely monogamous relationship. The risk of contracting or giving AIDS is otherwise too great.

• The best road to continued sexual health and pleasure is a healthy lifestyle. If we reduce our needs for medication (which we can), eat properly and reduce our body fat, increase our time at sensible but demanding physical activity, avoid or vastly temper our social use of legal drugs like alcohol, tobacco and caffeine and live a monogamous life, the other will follow if we dedicate ourselves to these goals.

• Either partner can start the engines.

ℰ Pause and Reflect

Aphrodisiacs, also called love potions, have been sought since the beginning of sex. Foods and herbs lead the list. Octopus, oysters and eels (they're all slimy) are still popular. Rhinoceros horns (looks like a penis), ground up, of course, goat glands sewn under the skin, garlic, pepper and ginseng root (they sting)—all these things and many, many more have been guaranteed as sexual enhancers. None of them are—but the placebo effect in this sexual area is about 50 percent! The FDA recognizes no over-the-counter preparation as a sexual stimulant. One formerly popular illegal agent, cantharidin or "Spanish fly," is an intense irritant to the lower urinary tract and sexual intercourse has, in this case, been compared to scratching an itch. Canthariadin overdose can be fatal.

The Hutterites are a very religious and moral sect that migrated into this country and Canada in the last century. They do not believe in birth control, and because they marry within their own ranks, they offer scientists an excellent opportunity to study declining fertility under natural circumstances and in a very healthy population. Studies indicate a marked and steady decrease in fertility after thirty in the Hutterites. In addition, the mean age of last live birth in this type of population preceded the menopause by about ten years.

Insofar as AIDS is concerned, the surest sexual way of transmitting it is by anal intercourse. This is not an uncommon sexual practice in our society; 238 of 723 women interviewed in 1987 about their sexual practices were active anal-intercourse participants. To protect yourself against AIDS you should avoid anal sex.

While on the subject of AIDS, this tragic condition is now very much a disease of women. One clinic reports that 31 percent of their new cases in the last three years have been from heterosexual contact and that 23 percent of their new cases were females. Besides the regular and terrible problems associated with this deadly disorder, women have two separate associated problems. They are subject to almost incurable yeast vaginitis and they are at much greater risk for premalignant and malignant disease of the cervix. Be sure that you understand that one (recurrent vaginitis and cervix disease) doesn't necessarily mean the other (AIDS). You will now find, however, that over-the-counter yeast preparations must carry an AIDS warning in their labeling.

———————

In the discussion on sexuality you learned that women's sex drive lasts well into the seventies and beyond. In one study, 20 percent of women interviewed at age seventy-five expressed continuing sexual interest. Most women with continuing sexual interest at this time of life weigh significantly more than the noninterested. It is believed that their extra fat stores more estrogen, which, in turn, stimulates sexual arousal.

———————

Sleeping and sleep disorders are very much more complicated than my short discussion would indicate. At least one-third of all Americans have some sort of sleeping problem. Over 40 million prescriptions are written each year for sleeping pills. Believe it or not, that represents a great reduction from the number written in a year a decade ago.

Modern sleeping pills, which are said to have a short half-life in the body, are now believed to have prolonged and sustained effects. The most important appears to be memory loss—something that often happens during the menopausal years and that doesn't need to be supplemented by drugs.

For more sleep information read *The American Medical Association Guide to Better Sleep,* by Lynne Lambert (Random House, 1984).

Men, here are some things to think about:

- Marriage may be the ultimate crucible, but it forges a pure human metal of great character. Men between forty-five and sixty-four who live alone are twice as likely to die within ten years as those men who live with their wives. Being sedentary, drinking, smoking, living with children or anyone else: Nothing altered this fact. Only living with a wife made the difference.

- There are 58 percent more men than women in mental institutions.

- Men lose their verbal abilities at a significantly earlier age than women.

- Twice as many women clean their belly button regularly than do men.

8

THE POSTMENOPAUSE
YEARS

This is your life—the *rest* of your life. And it could—and should—last a long time. Hopefully it will be free of the fetters that degenerative body changes can snare us with. We've talked about that.

These years lead us to our third life level—the Golden Years, Senior Citizenship and more. Actually, we become Master Citizens with all the rights and privileges. Thus we can backhand the government, get off useless committees, buy an occasional lottery ticket, park wherever, do our own thing and enjoy our quirks, straighten out our doctors and finally, enjoy being smarter than the next several hundred people.

So—what's our plan for this important one-third to one-half of life? What do we need to do—or continue to do—in order to delay and diminish anything that may inhibit our freedom till that very final countdown?

Here it is:

Hormone Replacement Therapy

Recall the four basic reasons for HRT:

- To protect and preserve sexuality.

- To delay or halt osteoporosis.

- To delay and diminish arteriosclerosis.

- To relieve flushes, sweats, insomnia and associated emotional changes.

Now then, flushes and sweats generally diminish on their own and are gone after a few years—even without HRT. The risk of both osteoporosis and arteriosclerosis, however, persists. Without HRT osteoporosis is very active for the first ten years or so following estrogen depletion, but it continues to melt bone forever. Arteriosclerosis, on the other hand, continues unabated. So do atrophy and thinning of the sexual organs along with diminishing sexual drive and capability.

It is clear, then, that HRT needs to be a continuing defense. Here are the principles:

- Provide the lowest effective dose.

- Stop menses if uterus is still in.

- Monitor carefully and regularly.

- Contain costs.

- Continue indefinitely.

The lowest effective estrogen dose appears to be .625 mg of oral estrone, 1 mg of oral estradiol or the smallest transdermal patch (0.05 mg).

The lowest effective dose of the commonest oral progestin (Provera) is 2.5 mg. Progestins are always used when the uterus is present. They promote regular cycles and protect against endometrial cancer. Commonly they are given 10–14 days in each cycle.

In the postmenopausal years it is desirable to eliminate the menstrual bleeding associated with *cyclic* HRT administration. This is accomplished by increasing the duration of progestin and estrogen administration so that eventually both hormones are taken on a constant daily basis. Menstruation ceases in the majority of women within six months.

Progestins have been accussed of unfavorably altering lipid (fat) levels in the blood but this has largely been disproved. Progestins do help estrogen protect bone and probably have other beneficial effects as well. See Chapter Five.

Testosterone

In the postmenopausal years, the ovaries continue to make small amounts of male hormone that may provide some sexual drive. Of course, if the ovaries have been surgically removed, there is no other significant internal source of testosterone. Often, under these and other circumstances, testosterone may be incorporated into a hormone program to stimulate and support sexual drive and orgasmic strength. The minimum oral dose would appear to be 1 or 2 mg daily.

Of course, critical care and control must be exercised in order to avoid unwanted side effects of testosterone (hair growth, voice change and acne, for instance) and to make certain there are no unwanted effects on bone and upon blood lipids. Most often, the minimum dose range has no unpleasant or harmful side effects, but your doctor will look for these possibilities.

Monitoring

Continuous and conscientious monitoring of these HRT programs is essential. That involves frequent (6–12 months) and regular doctor visits—your responsibility. It involves reporting unusual symptoms—your responsibility. It involves thorough consultation, examination, smears, mammograms, blood work, bone studies and any other indicated procedure or follow up—the doctor's responsibility. It involves consultation as needed, HRT adjustment and additional or supplemental medications as needed—the doctor's responsibility.

Cost Control

Generic estrogens are no longer available. Price-shop your prescriptions by phone. Mail-order pharmacies such as AARP and many insurance companies usually offer real savings. Ask that your prescriptions be written in full-bottle lots.

Quitting Time?

As yet there is no significant research to tell us that a certain cutoff age signals the time to end HRT. The proponents of HRT (of which I am one) feel that there is no single important and proper time to quit—barring, of course, the appearance of a substantial contraindication. Other less-eager menopausal managers suggest various cutoff points. Again, there is no scientific validation for either position. At this point, it appears to be an individual decision of patient and doctor based upon a number of equally individual factors. I feel that, as long as HRT continues to fulfill its protective role, it should be continued. Nothing has happened to my patients or in the field of research to alter that view.

The Cutting Edge

New preparations of estrogen and progesterone (and progestins) continue to be marketed.

- Pure oral micronized progesterone is becoming widely available. When progesterone has been used in the past, it had to be given by injection, by vaginal suppositories or by sublingual lozenges.

- Synthetic progestins are improving so that they mimic progesterone more closely.

- Newer low-dose oral estrogen pills will soon be marketed.

- Everyone knows about the highly successful under-the-skin (subcutaneous) birth control pellets that last five years. Are there similar long-lasting pellets of HRT on the market? Not yet. Estrogen and testosterone implants are available in some areas but their duration of action is short and that seems to be a hindrance to wider acceptance.

The Postmenopausal Lifestyle

To complement your HRT programs, you will want your lifestyle and habits to continue to be fully positive—just as in the menopausal years.

Exercise

Regardless of how good you feel and how hard you work at your health goals, aging is relentless. Thus, your heart output drops by 8 percent every ten years, your lung capacity decreases, your blood pressure tends to rise and your arteries get harder. Further, muscles weaken and joints stiffen, decreasing your mobility and power. Your bone mass decreases, even on HRT.

If you stay on your HRT program, all these aging problems are delayed—but you inevitably have to adjust to them. One way to adjust is through exercise. The basic philosophy of your post-menopausal physical exercise program is outlined in Chapter Six. The three main activity groups—aerobics, flexing and muscle strengthening—should all be continued, unless some physical problems intervenes and forces a shutdown. Continue your exercising at least three times weekly. You can do it.

Remember, walking, swimming and bicycling remain excellent aerobic exercises for you. Yoga may be a new way for you to increase flexibility and relaxation.

Remember the enemy: inertia, the tendency of a body to remain at rest. Keep moving!

Diet

The menopausal diet outlined in Chapter Six needs little alteration as you march along. There are a few changes as you age, however.

Your caloric intake must be gradually reduced since your needs will constantly decline. Most physicians agree that, depending upon your body frame and your activity level, you should aim for 1400–2200 calories daily. About 25 percent of this should be fat—proper fat.

Avoid highly seasoned foods. They become harder and harder to digest, so that after a four-alarm chili meal you may feel like you have just swallowed the world.

Decrease your intake of smoked foods and salty foods. Smoked foods increase your risk of cancer and salty foods increase your risk of high blood pressure.

Be sure you get your daily allotment of calcium and daily vitamins. Extra iron will not be so important if you are no longer menstruating and have no other blood loss disorder.

Include fiber in your meal. Reread the section about fiber foods and their different values in Chapter Six. Whole fresh fruits and vegetables are important and so is bran. And now there is evidence that even Metamucil will help lower your cholesterol level as well as supply you with safe, virtually calorie-free bulk.

Tobacco

If you continue to smoke, keep trying to break the habit. Every drag you avoid lengthens your life and the quality of it. Now, sad to say, is when the lifelong tobacco habit begins to round up its victims. Thus heart disease, strokes, emphysema and cancer—not only of the lungs but of many other body sites—begin their march across our lives. Stop smoking.

Alcohol

The abuse of alcohol is almost as deadly as the use of nicotine and tends to increase in women, for multiple reasons, in the postmenopausal years. Excellent help is available from AA and other support sources in almost every community. Meanwhile, a bottle of beer, a glass or two of wine or a drink of whiskey can be stimulating and relaxing—even healthful—to any of you who like alcohol and have no contraindicating health problems. Just don't offend or tempt nature or make a meal of alcohol.

Sleep

We talked about sleep somewhat in the last chapter. Recent studies indicate that as many as 80 million Americans suffer from some type of sleep disorder! It is, therefore, a large problem that has been largely ignored or neglected.

Sleep apnea, snoring and poor sleep quality are problems that increase with age and can have profound effects on our health—even leading to institutionalization in some cases. Sleep apnea (obstructed and delayed breathing), for instance, affects as many as 10 million Americans but no more than 5 percent of the apneics know they are so afflicted. This problem can lead to cardiovascular and cognitive complications—and even sudden death.

Your personal need for sleep doesn't change as time goes on. A number of things may waken you earlier and therefore you need to retire earlier. Try not to alter your normal sleep patterns and rituals and try to avoid naps.

Should you be concerned about a sleep problem, there are many registered sleep clinics in this country. For further help write:

> The National Sleep Foundation
> 122 South Robertson Blvd.
> Los Angeles, CA 90048

Medicine

Recent studies involving some 25,000 United States physicians (including me) strongly indicate that an aspirin tablet taken every other day reduces the risk of myocardial infarction (heart attack) by almost 50 percent! For five years, half of the participating doctors took a placebo and half took an aspirin every other day, none of us knowing what we were getting. The placebo group (which included me) had twice as many heart attacks. I'm now on aspirin.

Okay, so the study was done on 25,000 MALE doctors—now what about women? Well, this particular gender disparity has largely been overcome through research. The same positive effect of aspirin has been demonstrated in a much larger group of women. Not only that, aspirin has also been shown to significantly reduce the risk of colon and certain other gastrointestinal cancers. The cardiovascular protective effect is mediated by a reduction in blood coagulability, thus reducing the risk of clot formation in both the heart and the brain. The proven protective effect in gastrointestinal tumors is not clearly understood as yet.

In view of these positive findings, an aspirin (buffered if there are any stomach problems) every other day or a baby aspirin daily may very well fit into our postmenopausal arsenal. Some of us are allergic to aspirin or have other contraindications. Check with your own physician before embarking on this very protective (and cheap) program. And remember: MORE IS NOT BETTER.

Fulfillment

The firm base of friends and family that you have built will support you in all your encounters—good and bad—as your postmenopausal years unfold. There will be adversity through death, separation, divorce, illness, finances and loneliness. These temporal things can strike us at any time in our lives, but they multiply as we age. A lot of pleasurable and memorable things will also happen to us, so the good and the bad must be integrated and handled. Here is your plan:

Keep a circle of friends and keep interacting with them positively. A social network is a net that will catch you in a crisis.

Define meaningful goals for the future. Don't knit or do social, civic or community chores because you have nothing else to do. Do it because it is fulfilling for you—or do something else that is. There are thousands of things you can do.

When grief over a loss strikes you, let the natural grieving process unfold and run its course. Share your feelings with the various members of your network as they will share theirs with you. It helps. Speaking of help, it may be necessary, if grieving overwhelms you, to seek professional counseling. Don't delay accepting such help. There is no stigma attached to it.

It is important that you go back to Chapter Six and reread the Fulfillment section. Reaffirm the universal truth of a deeper, abiding and constant source of strength and power that surrounds us and is available to us just for the asking. Our human network can fail us—it is, after all, made up of us—but our spiritual power will not.

Continue to interact with your gynecologist/physician on a regular basis—at least once a year, preferably twice a year. Why?

- Your HRT needs to be constantly updated.

- Mammogram and bone density studies need reminding, reinforcement and monitoring.

- Regular Pap smears are important. Even with your uterus gone, you need a Pap smear every few years. With your uterus still in you need one every year, regardless of what you hear.

- A general physical examination with appropriate lab work will help you avoid degenerative changes, high blood pressure, heart disorders, serious gynecological disease and so on.

- Your doctor is—or should be—a part of your network as well as a counselor.

- This is a time when serious disorders of your pelvic organs are on the increase. Close and regular observation can only help in early detection and successful management.

Let's look at three malignancies of the pelvic organs that are more likely to appear in the postmenopausal years.

Cancer of the vulva appears as skin changes following aging and estrogen deprivation. Close observation and monitoring by modern colposcopic techniques can lead to treatment that can, in many cases, reverse, halt or correct such disorders before radical surgery must be undertaken to remove an actual cancer of the vulva.

Cancer of the endometrium is rarely seen before the menopause and usually many years afterwards. Again, close observation and biopsies at the slightest sign of postmenopausal bleeding help establish an early diagnosis. When endometrial cancer is diagnosed early, the arrest rates approach 95 percent. Moreover, many physicians are providing postmenopausal women with a provocative or challenge progesterone test every six to twelve months after the menses have ceased. In this test, a measured amount of progesterone (in the form of a progestin) is given over a week's time. In order for progesterone given as progestins to produce menstrual bleeding, there must be some activity in the uterine endometrial lining. Postmenopausally, if no estrogen is being administered, there should be absolutely no such endometrial activity at all. Thus, if the administration of a progestin does bring on any type of menstrual bleeding within a month after its administration, it must be assumed that some abnormal activity is present in the endometrium and that activity must be clearly identified by biopsy or by a D&C (dilatation and curettage) operation. As this challenge procedure becomes more widespread, it may allow the detection of early dangerous endometrial changes before they become invasive cancers. Remember that this same progesterone challenge test is also used to help determine the degree of ovarian failure in younger women. This has been described in Chapter Two.

Cancer of the ovaries is among the most feared of all female pelvic cancers but the outlook is improving. We'll talk about this malignancy in depth in Chapter Ten.

Bladder Problems

This is probably as good a time as any to bring up some of the unpleasant changes that commonly involve the lower urinary tract—actually the urethra more than the bladder. The urethra consists of a tube about two inches long that connects your bladder to the world. It is surrounded by a series of voluntary and involuntary muscles that—once you have become toilet-trained—will keep your bladder from emptying.

Two things happen in the postmenopausal years that affect the urethra:

- The muscles weaken—more so in women who have borne children. Thus voiding control becomes more difficult and unwanted leakage becomes more common—sometimes only on straining, sometimes anytime. Muscle strength can often be improved by a series of "Kegel" exercises (named for the man who first described the program). You can buy a pneumatic display monitor at your pharmacy that inserts into the vagina like a tampon and allows you to see your muscle strength improving. You will want to see a urologist to make sure that no other problem is involved in this loss of control. She will also give you Kegel exercise instructions—either orally or in a booklet form. Sometimes medications are helpful and, in certain cases of severe muscle damage, surgery may be indicated. HRT—taken orally or used locally—significantly helps delay muscle and urethral weakening.

- The urethral lining becomes thin and easily irritated and inflamed. Thus we have urethritis but not a true infection. There is a desire to empty more frequently and a burning at the end of urination. Chronic urethritis—the disorder's name—does not respond to antibiotics. It does respond to local treatments and to HRT. Actually it can generally be avoided or minimized with constant HRT—again locally or systemically. Prolonged, untreated chronic urethritis is usually accompanied by atrophic inflammatory changes in the vagina—called either atrophic or senile vaginitis. Both these conditions facilitate bacterial invasion and so true bladder infections (cystitis) are more common and more difficult to eradicate.

Thus we have two more conditions that respond to HRT and two more excellent reasons to continue it.

All in all, then, you need to put your doctor into your postmenopausal network program, interaction group or involvement program. Spend some quality time with her.

ℰ   Pause and Reflect

Postmenopausal women often experience a fractured wrist long before they begin to lose bone density in any significant amount. This accident appears to be a result of women putting out their hands to break a fall. Thus, evidence now points to the fact that, because of their increased postural sway, more menopausal women fall inadvertently, and that this particular fracture results from that fall, not from increased bone fragility.

_____

Recent evidence indicates that women on postmenopausal HRT have better long-term memories and greater concentration powers than their non-HRT sisters.

_____

Gender disparity in clinical medicine has been a hot topic in recent years—and rightly so. Although the National Institutes of Health has been instructed to include women in studies on an equal basis when applicable, little has been done. And in the practice of medicine, bias has been shown to exist against women in kidney dialysis and transplant, in the diagnosis of pulmonary cancer and in cardiac evaluation studies. On a more favorable note, there are 263 new medicines now being tested that are designed primarily for female problems.

Worldwide the incidence of depression is increasing at a regular and accelerating rate. Various reasons are given—longer lifespans (therefore more chronic illness), family breakups, the abuse of medications and drugs, social isolation, the waning influence of religion and more. Interestingly, light—natural or artificial—tends to alleviate depression and is now a common form of supplemental treatment. This would tend to explain the significantly higher incidence of depression in the winter. Humans deprived of light or in diminished light circumstances can rapidly become suicidal from depression.

A recent study, reported in the *New England Journal of Medicine,* revealed a tremendous dependency of Americans on unconventional forms of medication, such as acupuncture, massage, herbs, hypnosis, energy therapy, megavitamins and many more. The startling news was that an estimated 425 million annual visits were made to providers of these services at an out-of-pocket cost of $10.3 billion! This compares to out-of-pocket hospital costs of $12.8 billion during the same period.

9

ARTERIOSCLEROSIS AND OSTEOPOROSIS

We have already talked about both of these major disorders as our book has unfolded. However, they are such compelling and disastrous problems—and the mature years are when they haunt us most—that you will perhaps welcome some further reinforcement and understanding of them.

I'll try.

Arteriosclerosis

This disease is one of lifestyle—with a boost from genetics and, in women, with a boost from estrogen deprivation.

Excess circulating blood fats promote the formation of calcium plaques on arterial walls throughout the body. These plaques may eventually obstruct meaningful blood flow through the involved arteries and may also cause clots to form within the arterial channels themselves. Symptoms of such progressive

138

plaque-forming depend upon their location and size. Thus, the occlusion of even a small vessel in the heart or the brain is of great and immediate significance, whereas a similar-sized occlusion in the leg, for example, might go unnoticed. Numerous occlusions in the extremities, however, can cause great damage and loss of function. This is called peripheral vascular disease.

So cardiovascular disease marches on—fed by blood fats that come largely, but not exclusively, from our food.

Here's more:

- Cholesterol and triglycerides are the main blood fats (lipids). They are from two sources—our diet and our liver. If we got *none* of these fats in our diets—*none of them*—our livers could still make *all* we need!

- Blood fats are carried by blood lipoproteins since they are insoluble in blood itself. There are several lipoproteins but mainly high density (HDL) and low density (LDL) fractions are what concern us.

- HDL is apparently protective because it removes cholesterol from the circulation—the higher it is, the less likely coronary heart disease. It should measure greater than 35 mg per 100 ccs of blood—preferably about 65 mg in lipid blood samples. Lower than that may be related to a genetic disorder. No matter. The higher it is, the better.

- LDL should measure no more than 120 mg per 100 ccs in lipid blood samples. Absolute tops. LDL is apparently the dangerous lipoprotein, delivering cholesterol to the arterial walls. It also is influenced by genetic factors.

- Total blood cholesterol should always be under 200 mg per 100 ccs of blood. More than three-quarters of menopausal American women *exceed* that level!

- The above is a synopsis of a very complex biochemical lipid system. It only touches on the fringes of that system, but it is all we need to know.

Here are some other things we need to repeat about lipids:

- An American woman dies every sixty seconds from cardio-vascular disease. This mortality is twice that of *all forms of cancer*. Millions more are crippled by cardiovascular complications.

- Estrogen is cardioprotective. It lowers LDL and raises HDL. In the long run, progesterone affects neither HDL nor LDL.

- Because of the cardioprotective effect of estrogen, women rarely sustain heart attacks or strokes before the menopause. Afterwards, without estrogen, their risk mounts to exceed that of men. What is worse, they respond poorly to treatment and—even worse—may be passed over in treatment programs. Gender disparity.

- The benefits versus the risk of HRT—for this *one condition alone*—would seem to be a magnificent justification for its use.

- Certain other health and lifestyle factors markedly increase the cardiovascular risk. These include:

  - Cigarettes and other tobaccos.
  - Family history.
  - Obesity.
  - Hypertension.
  - Diabetes.
  - Sedentary lifestyle.

- History of previous cardiovascular accidents.
- Stress.

No matter what else is known, theorized, proposed, advanced or dismissed, the following lifestyle rules are vital to us.

- A sensible diet. No notepads or records needed—just eat right.

- No tobacco products. Modest red wine intake.

- Move the body—regularly and actively.

- Accept and follow proper management of diabetes, hypertension and obesity.

- Learn stress managment.

- HRT—of course.

This—or some other degenerative disorder—will collar us in the long run. No question about it. The game is to keep this particular disorder on the defensive as long as we can.

Osteoporosis

There is a similar onslaught from osteoporosis as the postmenopausal years gather steam. Actually, the condition begins to work its melting ways during the thirties, and it accelerates its erosion through the forties and the early postmenopausal years at an ever-accelerating rate, finally slowing down—but never stoping—about ten years after menses cease. All those events, of course, depend largely upon the absence of estrogen.

To give you just a glimpse into the magnitude of the osteoporosis cataclysm, here are some vital statistics:

- The disorder will eventually affect *every other* post-menopausal woman.

- One in three postmenopausal women will have a fracture sooner or later.

- There are in the United States 250,000 hip fractures in postmenopausal women each year. This will increase (unless we change our ways) to 500,000 by the end of this century.

- Of these women with hip fractures, 17 percent will die within three months, 40 percent within six months. Among survivors, 75 percent will lose their independence and 25 percent will require skilled nursing care.

- Eight out of every hundred women now thirty-five years old can expect to end up with a hip fracture sooner or later. Usually later. At least one-third of all women over ninety have sustained a hip fracture.

- Osteoporosis costs us about $10 billion now and will cost us over $30 billion by the year 2000 unless we change our ways.

- Twenty-five percent of all women over sixty have spinal compression fractures. This will rise to 50 percent before they are ninety.

The Bare Bone Facts

Physicians used to take great pride in exhibiting a full skeleton hanging prominently in their consultation rooms. The purpose of the skeleton was not very clear, but it did clearly reveal that the human frame was, indeed, made up of several hundred fairly uniform-looking bones that seemed very hard and unalterable.

Thus we all came away with the impression that the skeleton, made up of bones, was a fixed and permanent affair—much like the steel girders of a bridge.

Regardless of what we saw, however, our bony frame is not the least bit fixed and unalterable. It is a living and dynamic support system that is in constant change and that responds to many hundreds of variable stimulations, both good and bad, some building, some destroying. The commonest destroyer is osteoporosis, and it is second only to arthritis as the leading cause of disability among master citizens.

Here, then, is what you need to know about bone. Bone begins to form in embryos at about twelve weeks and continues to grow and develop for about twenty years. By that time our frame is generally complete and only the bone density may be altered.

There are two basic kinds of bone: cortical and trabecular. *Cortical* bone is the smooth exterior solid shaft that is visible on the surface of all bones. *Trabecular* bone is that found within the cortical sheath and is, in appearance, honey-combed. This very important bone functions like the small girders you see holding massive iron beams in place, keeping them from buckling. It is important to remember these two types of bone since they disappear at different times after the menopause.

Bone, under normal circumstances, is constantly being removed (by cells called osteoclasts) and constantly being rebuilt (by osteoblasts). This constant changing is called *remodeling*. Living bone is never at metabolic rest so it is constantly remodeling at an annual rate ranging from 50 percent in a two-year-old to 5 percent in an adult.

Normal and stable bone remodeling is controlled by many factors. Bone growth is stimulated by weight-bearing activity, sex hormones, pituitary growth hormones and normal thyroid activity. Bone loss is increased by physical inactivity, by excess adrenal hormones (corticosteroids) or thyroid hormones and by parathyroid activity, which is involved in calcium regulation, as well as by the absence of sex hormones, particularly estrogen.

Bone mass peaks between thirty and forty; proper diet and exercise will ensure that you have a maximum, stable, strong frame to carry you into the PMPX years.

As indicated above, women begin to experience bone loss in their thirties—even before menopausal symptoms develop. During the five to ten years that follow the menopause, a dramatic acceleration of bone loss begins—first the trabecular bone (which supports the vertebrae), and then, at a later date, the cortical bone. Thus, collapsed vertebrae, with the attendant pain and height loss, are usually the first clinical sign of osteoporosis.

One of the functions of bone is to store calcium for use when other bodily processes require it. These storage functions are regulated by certain cells of the thyroid glands, which secrete extra calcitonin when bone stores are being drained.

Let's look at an average person's daily calcium metabolism, remembering that this mineral needs to be kept in strict internal balance not only for bone strength but for all normal body functions.

Calcium comes into the body from dietary and supplementary sources. It leaves the body through the intestines and the kidneys. Obviously, for balance, the intake must equal the outgo. Each day the kidneys filter 8000 mg of calcium and lose 200 mg in the process. The intestines also lose another 300 mg of calcium each day. Thus, 500 mg of pure calcium must be absorbed from food and supplements each day to maintain balance.

Now then, to absorb 500 mg of pure calcium daily, it would be necessary to consume over 1000 mg of various calcium salts; but the average American diet provides only 650 mg. Thus, supplementation is almost always necessary—to the tune of at least 350 mg of pure calcium each day. Of the common supplementary calcium salts, calcium carbonate is 40 percent calcium, calcium lactate is 13 percent, calcium gluconate is 9 percent and calcium citrate is 30 percent calcium. Thus, if you use calcium carbonate (Tums, for instance) as your supplement, you would need to take at least 800 mg each day.

As suggested earlier, there are many categories of osteoporosis. They are classified as being primary or secondary. Primary osteoporosis includes both postmenopausal and age-related bone loss. Age-related loss affects both men and women as time goes on, but men lose bone much more slowly than do women. Postmenopausal osteoporosis, on the other hand, clearly affects only women and is very rapid. It is this type of osteoporosis that we will discuss here.

Secondary osteoporosis takes place when a specific disease or condition is responsible for skeletal bone erosion. Leukemia, hyperthyroidism (overactive thyroid), acromegaly (a problem stemming from the pituitary gland), rheumatoid arthritis, chronic lung disease and weightlessness (such as astronauts experience) will produce secondary osteoporosis in time.

Conditions that put certain women more at risk for osteoporosis include:

- *Genes and geography.* There are inherited characteristics for bone strength and weakness. Moreover, blacks are much less susceptible to osteoporosis than are Caucasian and Oriental women. Southern Europeans are more susceptible than their northern sisters.

- *Calcium deficiency.* Such deficiency may be due to inadequate calcium intake or to an inability to absorb calcium. This often occurs because of inadequate vitamin D intake.

- *Absent or inappropriate estrogen levels.* This is especially true in women who have lost their ovaries before the natural menopause.

- *Lack of regular, forceful exercise.*

- *Certain dietary aberrations.* Excess protein, caffeine, salt or alcohol may contribute to bone loss.

- *Tobacco.* Once again King Nicotine appears in the spoiler role.

- *Slight frame.* Thin women with small bones are at increased risk.

- *Childlessness.* Women who have never borne children seem to be at greater risk.

So if you are a short, thin, white, fair-complexioned lass approaching forty-five, and you sit on your can—indoors—all day, smoking, drinking alcohol and/or coffee, ingesting little or no calcium and failing to exercise—*watch out!* You are the perfect osteoporosis candidate.

The Diagnosis of Osteoporosis

Certainly our goal should be to prevent osteoporosis long, long before it becomes clinically evident, for osteoporosis is a silent thief, stealing bone for years before discovery. And restitution is just about impossible. We can barely catch the thief.

It therefore becomes important to anticipate the bone loss and to concentrate our preventive efforts upon those women at risk. This may involve some overactive and generous treatment, even among women who are not going to develop menopausal osteoporosis, but treatment does not involve increased risk if handled carefully.

Regular office examinations should include annual measurement of standing or sitting height plus the assessment of back pain and discomfort. Loss of sitting or standing height—particularly in association with acute or chronic back discomfort—is often the first clinical clue to this disorder.

Most of the pain associated with collapsing vertebrae from osteoporosis will eventually disappear since these fractures are stable in character and the vertebrae will adjust to their new condition. With a subsequent fracture, new pain will appear. Some dull chronic mid-back pain that responds to bed rest may persist between fracture episodes, but continuing severe pain would be suspicious of another disorder. Therefore, in the diagnostic workup, assessment of back structure and spinal cord health is important.

Laboratory Tests

Routine laboratory testing is almost useless in the detection of PMPX osteoporisis. Blood and urine levels of calcium generally stay within normal limits during osteoporosis, as do most other markers of bone destruction. In fact, normal laboratory tests simply help rule out other diseases that can cause bone disorders. Under clinical investigation are a number of as-yet-unproven laboratory tests to detect early osteoporosis. Thus, measurement of a certain pituitary hormone (GnRH), serum estrogen levels, urinary excretion of a certain group of body by-products and numerous other laboratory procedures are all under study. But none is yet ready to be used.

Imaging

There are several ways that picture-making can be useful, not only in making a diagnosis, but also in following the progression of osteoporosis. Imaging can also determine the bone's response to treatment. There are several types of imaging techniques:

- *X-rays.* Standard x-ray pictures of the skeleton will show collapsed, thin vertebrae along the backbone in advanced osteoporosis and will, of course, clearly show fractures. Yet x-rays cannot determine early loss of bone and so are not useful in the detection of osteoporosis.

- *Single photon absorptiometry (SPA).* This technique scans the wrist to see how much radiation from radioactive iodine is absorbed by the bones in that area. The radiation dose used is only 20 percent of that required for a chest x-ray. Although very precise, SPA measures primarily cortical bone, and so is not very useful in scanning the vertebrae or hips for trabecular bone loss.

- *Dual photon absorptiometry (DPA).* This technique involves the use of two photon beams of gadolinium. The rate at which these radioactive beams pass through the vertebrae or a hip bone will indicate, fairly accurately, the density of trabecular and cortical bone. As with SPA, there is little radiation exposure. Based on data supplied by DPA, it is possible to make fairly accurate predictions about future fracture risk.

- *Computerized axial tomography (CAT scan).* This technique, like DPA, measures radiation that passes through the bone. It has the distinct advantage of being able to separate trabecular from cortical bone. And it is very accurate. In a few areas of the United States, some special CAT scan equipment is individually designed for osteoporosis measurements. CAT scanning equipment is very expensive and usually hospital-based. In addition, the radiation exposure in a CAT scan is significantly greater than in other imaging techniques.

- *DEXA Imaging.* This is the very latest bone-imaging system. It is an x-ray technique that allows a reduced scanning time and provides very high resolution—both extremely desirable factors. The reduced exposure time is a safety net while the superior resolution gives us more accurate assessments of existing bone density and, perhaps equally important, allows for meaningful comparison pictures at shorter time intervals. DEXA imaging is generally available at this writing.

- Ultrasound and magnetic resonance imaging are not at this time in clinical use for bone scanning.

All in all, the dual photon procedure is the most widely used and the most acceptable clinical measurement of bone density. But even *without* bone scanning of any sort, *without* laboratory procedures and *without* much clinical study at all, the diagnosis of osteoporosis can be made and treatment instituted. Moreover, our major strategy today in taming this disorder is to prevent it from ever taking place.

The Treatment of Osteoporosis

As you have already guessed, the ideal treatment of osteoporosis is prevention and that is our real goal. Once bone is lost to this silent thief, it is difficult—some say impossible—to replace. It may actually be, however, that newer programs can replace some of the lost bone. It is clear though, that customary present-day therapy can only arrest bone loss; it certainly cannot fix already fractured and collapsed vertebrae. So prevention is the goal.

Many factors are important in controlling osteoporosis—diet, calcium, exercise, vitamin D, fluoride, avoidance of tobacco and alcohol and so on. But without estrogen, nothing else really works. So if prevention is the goal, estrogen is the road.

Hormone Replacement Therapy

HRT should be started as soon as internal production of estrogen diminishes to a symptomatic level (flushes, irregular menses, etc.) at the natural MPX or immediately after surgical removal of the ovaries in order to prevent osteoporosis. Of course, in every instance, there must be no valid contraindication to HRT. (See pages 55–57.)

Estrogen and progesterone should be given together for the following, already-stated reasons:

- Progesterone will protect the uterus against unilateral stimulation of estrogen, thus diminishing the risk of cancer of the endometrium.

- Many of us now believe progesterone has an equal protective effect against breast cancer. More believe it all the time but it is still not absolute.

- Estrogen retards bone loss, but it builds no new bone. Progesterone has been demonstrated to build new bone.

- By manipulating the dose of progesterone, it is usually possible to avoid menstruation in later years. Sixty-year-old patients are tired of carrying tampons in their purses.

HRT should be continued for at least ten years after the natural menopause, again to prevent osteoporosis. Many feel it should never be stopped—only reduced—as the years go by. Thus, if a woman sustains a surgical menopause at age thirty, for example, she should be supported by HRT for at least another thirty years. Unless something better comes along.

Diet

Most dietary habits involved in management of osteoporosis are noncontroversial, and most fall in line with your regular diet. (See pages 75–88.) The big controversy revolves around calcium—about which I could easily write a whole book. In general terms of diet, remember to avoid excesses of animal protein, caffeine, salt (any sodium, actually) and fiber.

Get as much dietary calcium as you can from food sources. Skim milk, low-fat yogurt, beans, cauliflower, broccoli, salmon, tofu and sardines are excellent sources, while most fruits, vegetables and cereals in your regular diet are good sources.

Don't drink more than two glasses of wine with your evening meal.

Calcium

For some time it was felt that adequate calcium intake alone could prevent osteoporosis. This is no longer a tenable theory. And rightly so. It is true that our average calcium intake is insufficient for our needs, but increased consumption alone is not enough.

American women take in about 650 mg of calcium daily. As you know, that isn't enough to maintain your daily calcium balance of 800 mg. Remember, that is 800 mg of pure calcium. The most common calcium supplement (calcium carbonate) is *less than* half calcium.

Most MPX women should have at least 1000 mg calcium daily—one way or another. Too much calcium is as bad as too little. Don't overdose.

Calcium levels in blood and other tissues must be kept constant. This regulation is managed by the parathyroid and thyroid glands. The thyroid gland secretes the hormone calcitonin, which is responsible for putting calcium back in bones when it's not needed for other bodily processes. However, low levels of calcitonin take calcium from bone to replace calcium not obtained from the diet. More on calcitonin later. The parathyroid glands, through their hormones, further fine-tune calcium blood levels.

The 1000–1500 mg suggested calcium intake does not increase your risk of calcium kidney stones or affect your medication for heart disease and high blood pressure (hypertension). In fact, it is becoming increasingly clear that an adequate dietary calcium intake protects against hypertension.

As you already know, estrogen has a protective effect upon bone and facilitates the absorption of calcium, thereby reducing its excretion via the kidneys.

So, what should your calcium program consist of?

- Eat a proper diet and you will get at least 650 mg calcium daily.

- Take about 400–500 mg more of pure calcium as a supplement. Two Tums, for instance, deliver 1000 mg of calcium carbonate (400 mg of calcium). Calcium carbonate (there are many other kinds of calcium supplements on the market) may be taken alone or with meals. Its only side effect may be constipation. Remember, don't overdose. More is not better.

- Include calcium citrate in your diet. Calcium citrate is becoming available on the market, both as a tablet and in certain fruit juices. It is absorbed more by the body more readily than any other form of calcium. Read labels for amounts and the available pure calcium.

- For maximum benefit, begin calcium supplementation early on. Remember, women begin to lose bone in their thirties due to inadequate calcium intake.

Exercise

Although there is no single, cleanly structured study that would prove the value of exercise in osteoporosis management, there is certainly a great deal of peripheral evidence. And, as you are aware, a regular exercise program has significant, progressive and prolonged value in your postmenopausal years.

If possible, it is important to build bone mass through diet and exercise before the menopause. Clear evidence indicates bone mass responds to repeated challenge. Thus, a tennis player may have as much as a 30 percent increase in bone mass in the racquet-holding arm! Other athletes show similar bone-growth responses. Conversely, bones rapidly demineralize in weightless individuals (such as astronauts).

As aging progresses and as falls become more ominous and more common, exercise is protective for two reasons: First, stability is improved and so falls are less likely to take place, and second, the increased mobility generated by regular exercise helps you "roll into" a fall and cushion its effect.

Incidentally, your home environment should eliminate as many "fall" traps as possible. Throw rugs, polished floors, loose steps and any other potentially dangerous articles should be banished.

Other Factors in Osteoporosis Control

VITAMIN D. This essential vitamin has several important roles in bone metabolism. It supports calcium absorption, slows calcium loss and promotes maintenance of the bone mass. Many food products (milk, for instance) have vitamin D added. Read the labels.

Vitamin D supplements are not necessary for women who are exposed to sunlight year-round. However, experts are now advising us to stay out of the sun because of the recent fearsome rise in a certain deadly type of skin cancer (melanoma). This cancer increase is attributed to overexposure to the heavier doses of ultraviolet rays now able to penetrate earth's polluted atmosphere.

Your daily intake of vitamin D need not exceed 600–800 international units. Overdosing with D can be very dangerous and will not help retain bone mass.

FLUORIDES. A very popular topic today. Fluorides will, in sufficient amounts, help build new bone, particularly trabecular bone. Whether they prevent bone loss is not clear. Therefore, the use of fluorides in osteoporosis must be considered experimental at this time.

If fluorides are used to treat osteoporosis, adequate amounts of calcium and vitamin D must also be given concurrently. Otherwise, serious bone disorders may follow.

Most urban water supplies in the United States now contain fluoride in varying amounts, mainly for prophylaxis (preventive benefits) against dental decay. The amount is very small, and its value in preventing osteoporosis at these levels is unknown.

Side effects of high fluoride dosage, such as leg cramps and skin rashes, occur in half the patients under study. The National Institutes of Health have several large-scale ongoing studies right now.

Don't try to get sodium fluoride on your own—yet.

CALCITONIN. Another hot item. You already know that calcitonin is secreted by the thyroid gland and that when the level of calcitonin circulating throughout the body decreases, it is a very important trigger in bone loss. Calcitonin has been used experimentally and is now FDA-approved for use in treating osteoporosis. However:

- It is very expensive and has to be given by injection or by nasal spray daily.

- There are often marked side effects of calcitonin administration.

- Calcitonin will not build new bone; it only slows the loss of old bone.

- Therapy with this drug should be reserved for severe osteoporosis that fails to respond to conventional lines of treatment.

- It is worth noting that both birth control pills and oral estrogens increase natural calcitonin levels.

DYAZIDE THERAPY. Dyazides, which are a group of diuretic (fluid control) medications, are now being used as a second-line treatment source for osteoporosis. These drugs promote the loss of water through the kidneys, and at the same time promote reabsorption of calcium, thus decreasing urinary calcium loss. There are, as always, potent side effects from dyazides, so they must be used with caution and only in patients with nonresponding osteoporosis.

Other treatments are in use here and there to manage osteoporosis. Testosterone, for instance—the hormone that athletes use to build bone and muscle mass—is clearly a positive force in building bone. It must, however, be balanced with estrogen and given with great care.

Experimental Osteoporosis Programs

Most osteoporosis studies involve attempts to build new bone or remodel existing bone structures. For instance, the use of calcitonin and oral phosphates to stimulate parathyroid activity and thus bone retention is one approach being studied at this time.

As an extension of the above experiments, a group of scientists are following up a cycle of parathyroid and phosphates with an additional two weeks of Didronel (etidronate disodium). This cycle of medication is repeated at regular intervals and the rate of new bone growth is very encouraging.

Human parathyroid hormone (HPTH), when administered along with a certain type of vitamin D, has been shown (in an experimental study group) to promote new bone growth. The study is continuing.

It is known that electrical field activity accelerates fracture healing. This technique is now being tried experimentally as a method of promoting new bone growth.

Other possible cures are too far down the line to even report upon. And all of a sudden, from a totally unexpected and unrelated source, the perfect treatment may appear. If you don't believe that's possible, read the story of the discovery of penicillin.

ℰ Pause and Reflect

Salmon is not only a good source of omega-3 fatty acids (see page 84), it is also rich in calcitonin. So, for that matter, are eels and lizards!

Most women who develop gouty arthritis (a condition in which crystallized substances are deposited within joint cavities, causing stiffness and pain) develop it after the menopause. Women receiving HRT, however, are apparently protected from gout and in one recent study, no woman on HRT could be found with the disorder.

Psychotropic drugs (tranquilizers) have been implicated in hip fractures among older women. With certain of these agents, the risk was increased up to 80 percent! Why? Most likely—although not certainly—because they caused increased instability and thus greater tendency to fall.

_____

Investigators are attempting to manufacture the proteins responsible for bone healing in fractures. They would then harvest such proteins and use them to promote new bone growth.

_____

Although exercise early on in life is very important in providing superior bone mass going into the menopause, can exercise be overdone? How do athletes fare in the MPX?

Many studies show that the average high school and college athlete does very well in the MPX, at least as well as her nonathletic counterpart. However, those women involved in strenuous, continued athletic competition—sufficient to induce amenorrhea and estrogen insufficiency—sustained bone loss of a significant degree in their vertebrae. What this will produce in later years is not yet known.

_____

Compared to currently married menopausal women, single, never-married women are over twice as likely to be hospitalized with a fractured hip, while divorced or widowed women are 1.7 times more likely to be hospitalized.

_____

Calcium from whole milk, chocolate milk, yogurt, imitation milk and pure calcium carbonate is absorbed equally well.

_____

Human hearts available for transplant are in short supply. Many patients will die awaiting suitable donor hearts. For instance, in America some 2,000 patients per month need new hearts but only about 100 are available. A report in the *Journal of the American Medical Association* (February 1993) describes a heart that sustained three people! It was donated to the first recipient who succumbed to some other complication. It was therefore removed and successfully implanted into its third owner.

Gene therapy is no longer confined to the science fiction domain. Altered genes are being reinserted into us at an ever-increasing rate for an ever-expanding number of conditions. Recently, altered genes were implanted into the liver of a woman who had a life-threatening inherited metabolic disorder that produced incredibly high blood cholesterol levels. The altered genes promptly began to manufacture liver cells capable of destroying circulating cholesterol. These altered genes were originally taken from her own liver cells and modified in the laboratory. Incredible!

10

BREASTS AND OVARIES IN THE MENOPAUSAL AND POSTMENOPAUSAL YEARS

t is strange and disturbing that a body part as lionized, talked about, photographed, painted, almost venerated, is as poorly understood insofar as disorders are concerned as the female breasts.

For example, cancer of the breast remains almost an enigma, while cancer of the lung is completely understood; the cause, the cure and the prevention are totally clear to us. Sadly, this cancer of the lung has overtaken cancer of the breast as the greatest malignant killer of women. This is not because breast cancer is decreasing, which it is not, but because lung cancer is increasing. This increase, of course, is based upon the increased number of women who began smoking at the end of World War II.

At any rate, we are just now beginning to understand the individual growth characteristics of breast cancer. It continues at the same occurrence rate or may gradually be increasing, and our treatment is no better—only slightly more humane and less mutilating.

Breast Physiology and Anatomy

In each female human breast, there are usually eighteen separate lobes. Each lobe contains glands that will secrete milk after childbirth, and ducts that will lead the milk to each nipple. Therefore, each nipple has eighteen separate ducts leading to it. This glandular and duct system is supported in a fibro-fatty network that holds everything in place. That, then, is the very basic architecture of each breast.

At the *thenarche*, which usually takes place from the ninth to eleventh year of childhood, the female breast tissue (which has been dormant) comes under the stimulation of a number of hormones—mainly estrogen, progesterone and human growth hormone. These substances promote growth and development of the breast, so that it becomes a mature organ capable of producing milk upon stimulation after obstetrical delivery.

Breasts also respond to other hormones. For instance, a pituitary hormone called *prolactin* is necessary for normal milk production. Incidentally, it also prevents menstruation. Thus, when a pituitary tumor of a certain type is present, excess prolactin is secreted and, even when no pregnancy exists, there will be secretion from the nipples (not milk, however) and absence of menstruation. This disorder is easily diagnosed but not so easily treated.

Other hormones secreted by the thyroid and adrenal glands affect breast growth and development, and another pituitary hormone, *oxytocin*, is responsible for the beginning of milk ejection during late labor and following delivery.

Of all these hormones, estrogen and progesterone have far and away the greatest effect on breast tissue. Estrogen is necessary for growth and development of the glandular tissue and progesterone is necessary for the maturation of many aspects of these tissues. As we move along in the study of breast disorders, we will see what effect these two hormones may or may not have.

Breast Disorders

Although there are many problems that can occur in breast tissue, ranging from simple infection during nursing all the way to cancer, there are three that occupy most of physicians' time and attention.

First, *cystic mastitis:* This is a very common disorder that results from the normal influence of estrogen and progesterone on the breast's glandular and duct structure. Usually it begins with unexplained duct obstruction, and as secretions back up behind the obstruction, tense, swollen gland tissue ensues. That in turn produces inflammation and tenderness. The end result is fibrosis, or scarring of local areas of breast tissue. Clinically, doctors can detect this condition when the breast tissue feels nodular and irregular in outline and has some firm areas of swelling and tenderness. Interestingly enough, as we will see later on, cystic mastitis tends to be less likely to occur in women who have been on oral contraceptives for a reasonably long period of time.

Cystic mastitis generally is characterized by breast pain, which may be intermittent in nature, may be worst just prior to periods and may be accompanied by nipple discharge. For some unknown reason, caffeine consumption apparently increases the irritation and pain of cystic mastitis. Whether cystic mastitis leads on to cancer or predisposes women to cancer is a hotly debated item. The consensus of present day thought is that it does not. Treatment consists of various hormone programs and caffeine restriction.

The second disorder is called *fibroadenoma*. Usually this condition develops in young women, but it also may occur at the perimenopause and even postmenopausally if hormone replacement therapy, particularly unopposed estrogen replacement therapy, is employed. Fibroadenomas, which are small, firm tumors present in the gland substance of one or more lobes, are caused by the *unilateral* stimulation of estrogen at any time in reproductive life. The problem is found more commonly in youngsters and in perimenopausal women because these individuals are usually not ovulating and thus not producing progesterone.

Fibroadenomas are benign tumors that may vary in size during menstrual cycles but will not disappear completely. They usually can be clearly defined by mammography. Generally no treatment is necessary, unless they cannot be clearly distinguished from breast cancer, at which time excision biopsy (complete removal of the growth at biopsy) is indicated.

The third breast disorder is *hyperplasia* (overgrowth) of gland and duct epithelium (lining cells). In this disorder, excess cells are formed in the surface layer of the milk-producing glands and ducts. This condition, which is very difficult to diagnose, is also apparently related to unilateral or unopposed estrogen stimulation. Both glandular and ductal hyperplasia are usually found when biopsies are performed for other, more obvious abnormalities in breast tissue. Symptoms are generally slight, and usually include a bloody discharge from the nipples. Very little or nothing can be felt in these cases. The only treatment is the administration of progesterone. The relationship of this condition to breast cancer is uncertain.

Nipple Secretions

After childbirth—without nursing or after nursing ceases—there will continue to be some secretion from the nipple—usually milky in nature. This secretion may persist for months but will gradually disappear—unless the breast is stimulated (lovemaking) or compressed. Some secretion regularly follows such stimulation but shortly stops.

Normal nipple secretions begin early in pregnancy and increase in amount as the pregnancy matures. Sometimes—because of the intense congestion of the breasts' glandular tissues during pregnancy—there may be an occasional tinge of blood in one nipple's secretions or in both. This somewhat unsettling, though natural phenomenon, disappears after delivery.

Other than the above circumstances, nipple discharges are considered abnormal and should be investigated.

Here's more information:

- Discharges from one breast only are most worrisome—particularly if they are watery or blood-tinged.

- Constant milky leakage from both nipples is usually due to excess prolactin secretion from the pituitary gland (see page 160). This can usually be corrected.

- Greenish or brown discharges that can stain bras are usually related to inflammatory conditions in the ducts.

- If actual pus is present in the discharge, it is usually due to an infection and some area of the breast will probably be red, swollen and tender. It should disappear with appropriate antibiotic therapy.

- Abnormal secretions are more likely to be associated with cancer in older women. Most often 85 percent of all discharges are associated with benign conditions.

No matter what the discharge type, all need to be investigated. Studies may include cytology (a sort of breast Pap smear), bacterial cultures, mammograms, ultrasound, injecting ducts for x-ray studies (ductography), hormone studies and biopsies.

Cancer of the Breast

The enormity of this disorder cannot be overstated. Although cancer of the lung now destroys more women than does breast cancer, it is only because the former is increasing and not because breast cancer is decreasing. Here are some more things you may want to know:

- The news is now widely disseminated that breast cancer will strike one woman in nine during her lifetime. This statement needs to be clarified. What it REALLY MEANS is that, if she lives to be eighty-five or more, her chances of developing breast cancer would indeed be one in nine. But at twenty-five her chances are 1:20,000; at forty, 1:217; at sixty, 1:24; and so on up the age scale. Incidentally, the maximum life expectancy rate in these statistical studies has been raised to ninety-five. At that age, the risk is 1:8.

- Thus, the chances are increasing because women are living longer. Similarly, if men live long enough, the majority of them will get prostate cancer.

- The actual breast cancer RATE in this country has fallen for the second straight year—from 109.6 cases per 100,000 women in 1988 to 104.6 in 1989. No later figures are as yet available. So—you see what figures can do!

- More figures, though. Breast cancer starts from a single abnormal cell—almost always. This, of course, multiplies as time goes by. It takes SEVEN YEARS to reach 1 millimeter in size. For comparison, there are about 25 millimeters in one inch; one millimeter is about the size of a pinhead. This is about the time that it will first appear on a mammogram. In two to three more years the tumor has grown to about one centimeter and can usually now be felt—but not always. Mammograms, then, give us a two-year treatment window even though they are not perfect.

- Most of these growths (50 percent) occur in the upper outer breast quadrant. The rest may be found anywhere in breast tissue.

- Recent understanding of this disease's nature has greatly altered the treatment. It is now considered a more-or-less systemic disorder early on and thus extensive local destructive treatment has given way to more comprehensive systemic therapy.

- As a result of the newer understanding—and earlier diagnosis—survival rates are at last improving significantly. Moreover, there is less mutilation of breasts due to surgery.

- Although the chances of acquiring breast cancer increase with age, still most actual cases are seen in and around the menopausal years. That's because there are more women living in that age group. Fortunately, treatment seems to be more successful at this time in life.

Who Is at Greatest Risk for Developing Breast Cancer?

The following factors determine who is most likely to develop breast cancer:

- *Family history*. Women whose family history includes female relatives who have had breast cancer have a significantly greater risk, particularly if these relatives are on the maternal side, and particularly if their breast cancer developed earlier in life (before the menopause). The closer the family link, the longer the risk lasts. For instance, if the positive occurrence of breast cancer in the family history involves an aunt or grandmother, the increased risk is until sixty. If, however, the link is a mother or a sister, the risk extends to sixty-five.

- *Age at menopause*. The later the menopause begins, the greater the risk of developing breast cancer. This may be related to prolonged unopposed estrogen production after ovulation ceases.

- *Pregnancy.* Pregnancy exerts, probably through hormonal patterns, a protective influence against the development of breast cancer. The earlier the pregnancies occur, the greater the protection. Thus, women who have never borne children are at a greater risk for breast cancer.

- *Ovarian activity.* Women with prolonged anovulatory cycles (periods of time during which ovulation does not occur), that is, who are exposed to unopposed estrogen over the years, are at greater risk.

- *Nutrition.* Women who are obese, women who are diabetic and women who are on a high-cholesterol diet are more susceptible to breast cancer. This again is related to the production and storage (in fat) of unopposed estrogen. Also on a nutritional basis, there is now evidence that alcohol consumption increases the risk of breast cancer. It is important to point out here that the data upon which this conclusion is based are recent and not clearly established. However, this is something that bears further study.

- *Ethnic background.* It is clear that some ethnic groups are at greater risk of developing breast cancer. Thus, North American and Western European women are at significantly greater risk than are Japanese, black and Indian women. Moreover, women in an upper socioeconomic level are at greater risk. This may be related to many factors that are not directly involved with social background.

- *Previous breast cancer in one of the breasts.* This clearly increases the risk of recurrence in both breasts. There is now considerable controversy among experts in the field, some suggesting that after cancerous breast tissue is removed, removal of the other breast (along with plastic reconstruction of both breasts) may be a wise procedure. More on this later.

- *Other factors*. Previous multiple chest x-rays, marital status, country versus city living and so forth also play some role in the genesis of this disorder.

The Diagnosis of Breast Cancer

Many techniques have been employed in order to facilitate and speed up the diagnosis of breast cancer. It is very clear that the earlier the diagnosis is made, the more successful treatment will be and the greater the quality of life in the survivor. There are three basic methods of diagnosis.

Breast Self-Examination

Although considered an anachronism by many scientists, it still remains the most productive method of detecting breast cancer today: 90 percent of all breast cancers are discovered by breast self-examination. It has been shown that women who are unskilled at breast self-examination cannot detect a tumor until it is at least *twice* the size of a tumor that a more skilled woman could identify. The technique is explained in many of the free pamphlets published and distributed widely by the American Cancer Society. (Write to the American Cancer Society, 90 Park Avenue, New York, NY 10016, and they will be happy to send you an outline.) In addition, many physicians have pamphlets in their offices describing the technique for breast self-examination and breast cancer detection centers teach and encourage this form of examination.

In many instances, husbands become skilled supplemental breast examiners, and they should be encouraged to do this regardless of what sexual overtones can be read into it. I advise you to learn breast self-examination. During the first year of self-examination your breasts may feel lumpy, irregular and filled with disease, but you will eventually come to know the topography and architecture of your breasts very well.

Physician Breast Examination

Regular palpation of breast tissue by your physician should be a part of your annual examination. Under certain circumstances, more frequent examinations are clearly indicated. Your physician's examination may be different from your own examination, but the same structural abnormalities are being sought after. You should be willing, indeed anxious, to have your physician examine your breasts, and he or she should be equally anxious to do so for you. Again, early detection is vitally important and you and your physician together can do a better job than either one alone. Persistent breast masses should be identified and diagnosed to everybody's satisfaction.

Imaging Techniques

These diagnostic procedures are far and away the most important methods available today in making an early diagnosis of breast cancer. The techniques used today include mammography, ultrasound and magnetic resonance imaging.

MAMMOGRAPHY. Of all the imaging techniques, nothing at this time approaches the mammogram in its efficiency in determining the presence or absence of breast lesions and identifying their malignant or nonmalignant characters. Here are some very salient points about mammography:

- Although not 100 percent successful in finding breast cancer, mammography has the lowest failure rate of any known technique today. It will often detect a tumor as many as two or more years before it could have been felt either by the woman or her physician.

- All mammograms involve the use of x-rays. Mammogram exposure rates, insofar as radiation risks are concerned, are minimal, however. Assuming a patient had twenty mammograms in a lifetime, her radiation exposure risks in terms of developing cancer would be equivalent to smoking *four* or *five* cigarettes in a *lifetime*. This would appear to be a very acceptable risk.

- Mammogram screening clinics are springing up everywhere in the United States. Screening mammograms are done in every kind of setting—x-ray offices, doctors' offices, mobile clinics, shopping malls—anywhere a certified technician with the proper equipment can set up shop. They are taken as a routine age-based screen and are not taken when disease is present or suspected. Under those circumstances a mammogram is diagnostic and is performed at a radiology clinic only. Screening clinics are increasing the availability of this technique and, by and large, decreasing the cost. As an example, there are four mammographic screening clinics in the Little Rock area. These clinics, which generally operate on a walk-in basis, charge $65 for a mammogram and an explanation of breast self-examination. In some places, a mammogram can cost up to $300, but competition is rapidly eliminating such elitist institutions. Mammograms should be read by certified radiologists, preferably ones who have received added training in the interpretation of mammograms. This is true even for screening mammograms.

- Most mammographic examinations nowadays are performed with equipment used ONLY for this one purpose. They are called "dedicated." Moreover, the technicians who take your mammograms and the radiologist who reads them are generally especially certified to do these important tasks. Notice of such certification is often posted for all to see.

Mammograms are most useful among women of the age groups most likely to develop breast cancer. Thus the general recommendation for screening is as follows:

- First screening at thirty-five, also known as "baseline."

- Repeat every two years starting at forty.

- Repeat annually at fifty for the rest of life.

These suggested intervals and times change, of course, if a breast lesion is found. They also change if there is a family history of the disease—particularly if the relationship is close and the onset early in life. Your physician would advise you.

There is now some confusion and disagreement surrounding the screening intervals spelled out above. This state of affairs is largely due to a recent Canadian study that apparently showed no reduction in breast cancer mortality among women in the forty–fifty age group who had regular mammograms compared to those same-aged women who did not. The thrust of the study, then, was that mammograms in the forty–fifty age group were of no value. For a number of reasons, the study has been widely criticized and in the United States, almost every responsible group recommends continuation of our regular screening program. Indeed, the Radiological Society of North America, meeting in January 1993, recommended that no change be made in the American screening programs.

- Most states now mandate that insurance companies include regular mammograms in their insurance coverage. Medicare covers mammograms in their own peculiar way and to a certain amount. The coverage by both insurance and Medicare varies widely, changes constantly and cannot be outlined here.

- Mammograms are not perfect. The general false negative rate (missing a tumor) is around 10 percent. And the false positive rate (seeing something when nothing dangerous is there) is around 2 percent. Nevertheless, nothing—NOTHING—comes close to this test at this time as an early marker for breast cancer.

- The number of women who ever had a mammogram has increased significantly (74 percent). This increase has been among white women of higher education and incomes. Of these women, 76 percent did it because of physician recommendation. Physicians—all of us—however, are not doing as well as we could in pushing our patients into continuing screening programs. This includes laboratory and self-examinations.

ULTRASOUND IMAGING. This is a very safe, noninvasive imaging system that assists us in refining mammographic findings. Generally, ultrasound is not used as an initial screening device. However, when a nodule or a suspicious area on the breast is identified, the ultrasound further clarifies its identity in two ways.

- It provides great help in determining if a previously visualized growth is solid or cystic. Such a determination can make a tremendous difference in treatment. Cystic growths are much more likely to be benign.

- New "doppler" ultrasound can determine blood flow patterns in arteries and veins. Such information is of great importance in treating a number of disorders. There are many other valuable uses of doppler flow tests. For instance, they tell us about blood flow to the brain through the carotid arteries when we suspect that brain circulation may be diminished. In breast cancer detection, doppler studies of an already-detected lump can help us determine blood-flow patterns through that lump. Such patterns usually have characteristic differences when a malignancy threatens. Doppler flow studies are not yet universally available.

MAGNETIC RESONANCE IMAGING (MRI). This fantastic, very expensive, very safe imaging technique has become generally available in America. But its role in breast imaging is limited for two reasons:

- It's too expensive as a screening tool.
- As yet it can't be shown to beat the accuracy of x-ray mammography.

Currently, then, its use is investigational and perhaps as a follow-up for cases of previous breast cancer that have been treated with large doses of radiation. MRI may be the wave of the future, but other techniques and equipment, using entirely different approaches, are likely to supplant anything now available to us.

THERMOGRAPHY AND TRANSILLUMINATION. These procedures involve analysis of the radiation of heat from breast tissue or the transillumination of light through it. Tumors radiate more heat than healthy tissue and block the transmission of light. Neither method appears to be very accurate, even for minor screening techniques. Therefore, neither is widely recommended.

FINE NEEDLE ASPIRATION (FNA). Before leaving diagnostic procedures, some mention of FNA is necessary. After a breast lesion has been identified by imaging or by feeling, it is not uncommon to do a FNA procedure. What is involved here? Well, first, it is an office procedure. Under local anesthesia, a fine needle is inserted into the lump and material withdrawn from it. This material is analyzed by a pathologist and, if negative, no further studies are carried out. However, close follow-up on a continuous basis is necessary.

FNA has reduced the number of biopsy breast surgeries performed and has a growing number of proponents. It is still a disputed technique and so your personal physician may not want to do it. But you will hear more about it. The popular press will be writing about FNA, and should you have any breast problem whatsoever, your breast surgeon will very likely discuss this procedure with you.

FNA must not be confused with open wire biopsy. This method involves insertion of a wire (through a needle) by a radiologist under direct imaging. The patient then goes to surgery and under anesthesia the surgeon follows the wire down to the lesion and removes the tissue around it. This, then, is a hospital procedure and considerably more involved. Further, it may well be curative as well as diagnostic.

The Treatment of Breast Cancer

This is a very complicated and complex subject that we cannot begin to cover in this menopause handbook. Basically, the treatment will vary significantly depending on whether the patient is premenopausal or postmenopausal and whether or not the lymph nodes in the armpits test positive for cancer cells. Again, there appears to be less emphasis today on radical local surgery and more upon local excision of tumor mass and more generalized body treatment with radiation and/or chemotherapy. Should you, God forbid, be diagnosed as having a breast malignancy, you should consider consulting two competent breast surgeons before submitting to any therapy.

HRT and Breast Cancer

As you already know, hormone replacement therapy involving proper combinations of estrogen and progesterone does not cause cancer of the endometrium, and in fact protects the endometrium against the development of malignancies. Since breast tissue contains target cells affected by estrogen and progesterone, won't the combination of estrogen and progesterone protect this tissue against the ultimate development of breast cancer? Although there is still considerable argument among investigative scientists in this regard, it is becoming clear that estrogen and progesterone (progestin) given in proper combinations will protect the breasts against the development of cancer. The evidence is as follows:

- Women who have been on long-term oral contraceptives (which are a combination of synthetic estrogen and progestins) have been conclusively shown to have less risk of breast cancer than women who have not taken oral contraceptives. A thorough review of all of the literature on oral contraceptives refutes the view that they increase the risk of breast cancer.

- Women who develop breast cancer and formerly used birth control pills have a greater overall survival rate than those breast cancer patients who never used birth control pills.

- The largest studies accumulated to date on the use of HRT in menopausal and postmenopausal women clearly show that the breast is protected against cancer by the use of combined estrogen and progesterone replacement therapy. The use of estrogen alone appears to be nonprotective but has not clearly been perceived to be dangerous.

- When progestational agents are experimentally added to cultures of human breast cancer cells, the multiplication of cancer cells is inhibited.

- Premenopausal women who undergo breast surgery in the progestational (second) phase of their menstrual cycle have a significantly longer arrest time.

- Large doses of progestins are being used to treat breast cancer.

Thus, it is evident that in the absence of an existing breast cancer, appropriately given hormone replacement therapy will protect the human female breasts against the development of cancer. It is becoming clear, however, that progestin compounds should be included in such HRT therapy.

Tamoxifen (Nolvadex)

This agent is now being widely used as an addition to our therapies for breast cancer. It is also now involved in a very large study, sponsored by the government, to see if it can prevent breast cancer. More on that in a moment.

Here are some points about Tamoxifen:

- It resembles stilbesterol—a synthetic estrogen-like drug that caused a great deal of problems in the past. Although it is too early, to tell for certain, Tamoxifen does not appear to carry any of stilbestrol's long-term problems.

- Tamoxifen was originally thought to be a potential birth control pill but was not sufficiently dependable.

- It is an antiestrogen in that it competes and displaces estrogen from potential receptor sites. Thus estrogen effects are diminished. This is termed estrogen-receptor-positive.

- Tamoxifen therapy, therefore, is fully justified in postmenopausal women with estrogen-receptor-positive breast disease. It also appears of value in early breast cancer regardless of receptor status.

- The drug seems to stop tumor cells from growing rather than killing them. Therefore it must be used continuously for an indeterminant number of years.

- Disease-free survival time is increased and total survival time increased from 20 to 75 percent with Tamoxifen, depending on a number of factors including age, initial stage of disease and receptor status.

- Tamoxifen is given orally—usually 20 mg daily. It can cause significant nausea and vomiting in a few patients. Other side effects include eye irritation and weight gain. It also can cause menopausal symptoms—flushes, sweats, dry vaginas, etc. In one study, frequent simple ovarian cysts were a problem.

- Some unexpected effects of Tamoxifen include:

  - Continued bone protection.

  - Unchanged blood lipids.

  - Stimulation of the endometrium in postmenopausal women. Bleeding may begin and endometrial biopsies may be required. A few cases of endometrial cancer have been reported.

The experimental long-term use of Tamoxifen in breast cancer prevention involves some 16,000 women. Half will receive the drug, half will receive a placebo. All the women selected have a history of increased risk for breast cancer. The study is designed to last five years but may be extended or shortened, depending upon a number of unknowns such as early good results or serious unexpected side effects.

Many arguments are being raised against this study—the risk of birth defects if pregnancy occurs; the risk of producing Tamoxifen-resistant breast tumors; the risk of inducing endometrial cancer; potential side effects, some as yet unknown; and so on.

The NIH responds by saying that this trial is one of the most important ever undertaken in regard to female health. It is believed that the drug may reduce breast cancer by one-third.

We all certainly hope so.

HRT Following Breast Cancer

For a number of reasons, it has become appropriate to consider the institution of hormone replacement therapy in women who have undergone adequate therapy for cancer of the breast. This is particularly true in young women who have had breast cancer and who are having significant menopausal problems. Severe flushes, depression and vaginal atrophy with painful intercourse are examples.

Since many breast cancers are "estrogen dependent" and thus grow more readily in its presence, hormone replacement therapy can be considered only in cases where the breast tumor was discovered very early and when there has been evidence of complete arrest for at least five years. Although there is not a large body of research available in this area, more and more data supporting HRT after breast cancer are accumulated as each year goes by. Research is limited by the risks of malpractice, the dogmas of prior teaching authorities and prior theories and by clearly understandable patient fears. Yet many patients, having been thoroughly informed about the risks and benefits of hormonal replacement therapy following five years of cancer arrest, are now accepting HRT. The safety of such programs cannot, of course, be documented for many years to come.

Let me end this disheartening section on breast cancer with what I feel is a great coming breakthrough in the treatment of all cancers.

Immunologists, using monoclonal antibody technology (which is too complex to explain and not necessary to explain for our needs anyway), can now make immune proteins for specific cancers. These can then be "radiolabeled" with minute amounts of radioactivity. Injected into the bloodstream, these immune antibodies attach at once to any such cancer cells in the body. Screening the body now will identify if cancer is present and give a clear picture of its extent and/or spread. Thus, if breast cancer antibodies are injected and there are no breast cancer cells present, screening of the breast tissue for radioactivity will reveal none and so the test will be negative. If, on the other hand, a breast cancer exists, it will be found, no matter how small, and screening will tell its extent and location clearly, and any spread will be visualized as well—a marvelous diagnostic tool. But there is more.

Using the same monoclonal antibodies—this time made highly radioactive—we can thus inject a cancer killer that will go directly to the tumor cells no matter where they are, grab hold and go nowhere else!

There is still much to be done, but investigators feel this technique will be in use in this century.

The Ovaries

We have been deeply involved with the life-cycle of these incredibly complex reproductive glands since the beginning of our book (some of us since the beginning of life!). Because of their very diverse cellular architecture, many equally diverse problems may develop within them.

There are two main cell types within the ovaries. "Germinal" cells are those capable of maturing into eggs and of producing hormones during reproductive life. Germinal cells are enmeshed in "epithelial" cells, which bind the ovaries together and which themselves may have some hormonal production potential. Germinal cells are found only in the ovaries while epithelial cells of various types are found almost everywhere in our bodies.

During active reproductive life, benign cysts are, of course, a monthly event and persistent, often large cysts are not unusual.

Moreover, because of the multipotential germinal cells that lie within, certain bizarre, often fatal tumors may rarely occur—even in youngsters.

It is during and after the menopause—when ovarian activity has ceased for the most part—that concerns rise sharply for epithelial ovarian cancer. This is the major ovarian tumor, attacking some 21,000 American women each year (producing a lifetime incident rate of 1:70—though remember from breast statistics, "rate" can be misleading). Because of late diagnosis, this treacherous cancer has a poor survival rate.

Here are some more facts about ovarian cancer:

- Oral contraceptives provide very significant and prolonged protection against this cancer. The more years on the pill, the better the protection—and the longer that protection lasts once the pill is discontinued.

- Identified risk factors include having had no children or few children, early menarche, late menopause, late first pregnancy and family history. The last—family history—is the only substantial risk factor. More on that in a moment.

- Recently, several studies have suggested that the use of talcum powder as a perineal hygienic measure increases the risk of ovarian cancer! The belief is that talc migrates up the reproductive tract and acts as an ovarian irritant. Strange as it may seem as a source of ovarian cancer, some authorities nevertheless advise discontinuance of this practice.

DETECTION. Because ovarian tumors grow in a relatively inaccessible area and produce no symptoms early on, they are usually diagnosed late and thus the poor survival rate. Naturally, then, a great deal of energy is being devoted to better screening and diagnostic tests. Progress is slow but picking up.

- Regular pelvic examination. No matter how good and thorough the examiner, no matter how often it is done, no matter how thin and cooperative the lady, pelvic examination is of little value as a screening device for ovarian cancer. The examination does provide continuous physician contact, however, and makes the likelihood of further screening procedures more real. Don't avoid doctor contact—routine gynecological examinations reveal a host of other problems that could be equally threatening.

- Ultrasound. Transabdominal ultrasound is not much better than a pelvic examination as a screening tool for this tumor. Transvaginal ultrasound is considerably better and transvaginal doppler (look back to breast screening) ultrasound refines this procedure even more. Some doctors are using this combination as a screening tool, but by itself there is still an unacceptably high rate of false positives.

- Serum tumor markers. Tumors in the body produce chemical changes that act as "antigens" and are picked up by the bloodstream. Samples of blood that contain these antigens can be detected and measured by "antibodies" against the tumors. These antibodies—called serum tumor markers—are manufactured in the laboratory by very complex molecular chemistry but are becoming readily available as a diagnostic tool. One of these, for instance, called PSA (prostate specific antigen) screens very well for male prostate cancer. Another is now being studied as a screen for colon cancer and a third—CA-125—is widely used in screening for ovarian cancer and for following treatment goals in managing this cancer. Certain body disorders (endometriosis, for instance) can produce moderately low levels of CA-125 but if levels rise above 35 units per cc of blood, cancer of the ovary must be considered. This is particularly true if subsequent CA-125 levels continue to rise. So CA-125 levels are not now absolutely specific for ovarian cancer, and other tumor markers—called CA-15-3 and TAG-72.3—that hold promise for more specificity are now being studied. The growing literature on tumor marker investigation—just now beginning to mature—reads like science fiction.

- Fine needle aspiration (just as in the breast)—either transabdominally or transvaginally—from a pelvic mass is used as a diagnostic tool in some centers.

Now, in order for a screening procedure to be acceptable, it must meet certain standards.

- It must be highly sensitive and specific. For instance, an ovarian cancer test that was 99.6 percent effective would mean ten patients would have to undergo surgery to find one ovarian malignancy!

- It would have to be cost-effective.

- It would have to reduce mortality.

The combination of advanced transvaginal ultrasound using doppler assist, along with CA-125 screening, might fulfill two of the above three requirements. It would, however, cost $14 billion a year to institute. That is not considered cost-effective.

We are left then with no acceptable screening tools or combination of screening tools at this time. It is likely that monoclonal antibody screening will soon be sensitive enough for us to use as a screening procedure—and, with some modifications, even as a treatment tool. Please read in the breast section what I said about this anticipated breakthrough. See page 177.

FAMILIAL OVARIAN CANCER. The tragic loss of Gilda Radner in 1989 from ovarian cancer that had a familial background has had at least three positive effects. It has created a wealth of information for the Familial Ovarian Cancer Registry, which now bears her name; it has stimulated research and study in this tragic area, and it has certainly heightened physician-patient awareness of the inherited potential of this cancer.

There are three categories of familial ovarian cancer:

- A familial history of ovarian cancer alone.

- A cluster of both ovarian and breast cancer in these families.

- Cancer family syndrome—not only ovarian cancer but cancers of the colon, lung and prostate as well.

Women who have two first-degree relatives with ovarian cancer have a 50 percent chance of developing the disease and often develop it early in life. With one first-degree relative only, the risk is considerably less (20 percent).

The consensus among doctors for managing this group of women is as follows, remembering there are also wide variations from the consensus.

- Birth control pills represent an extremely safe, long-term protective medication and as such, should be considered whenever possible, as early as possible (once menstrual function is well established) and for as long as possible.

- Regular screening with the techniques we have talked about should be part of their routine examinations. In these families, the tests are justified and cost-effective. They should be undertaken early on—even in the late twenties.

- Protective removal of the ovaries should be strongly considered by women at high risk. This—as you might imagine—is a hotly debated topic. Here are some points:

- At-risk women about to undergo a hysterectomy should be encouraged to have this protective ovarian removal.

- The ovarian cancer rate would be reduced in this cluster by 50 percent, the total rate by 15 percent.

- Ovary-like cancer could still occur, though rarely, from peritoneal (abdominal-lining) cells that are embryologically similar to ovarian cells.

- The potential risk of subsequent HRT in this sensitive group would need to be considered—particularly in the second and third familial categories.

As you can see, malignant ovarian disease is a very complex disorder and there are wide divergencies among the experts concerning the various diagnostic and treatment programs that exist today.

The treatment is equally complex and too diverse and variable for us to cover. Our first hope is improved, consistent and early diagnosis along with the preventive measures that we have already talked about.

The latest treatment drug—Taxol—is making a splash in the press. It is derived from western Pacific yew trees. One course requires the bark from four to six one hundred-year-old trees and the cost is enormous—to the patient and to the environment. Someday it will be synthesized but perhaps much better treatment is really closer at hand.

ℰ Pause and Reflect

As a part of sex-change therapy, genetic-true males who are being converted into females are given large doses of estrogen that will produce enlargement of the breasts. No progesterone or progestins are given. There are now *two* reported cases of breast cancer among such genetic males receiving estrogen therapy. This does not speak well for the way breast tissue responds to unopposed estrogen.

––––––––––

Women whose breasts have been augmented by surgical procedures (implanted prosthetic devices) can still be studied properly by routine mammographic examinations. Such examinations are, however, much more difficult to interpret.

––––––––––

Some evidence exists that women who have pacemakers inserted in the chest wall should undergo more frequent mammographic examinations. One study has revealed a threefold increase in breast cancer on the side in which a pacemaker has been implanted. Although this particular subject might now be debated, it still should not be overlooked.

––––––––––

In 1992, then–President Bush signed into law two important medical bills. First, the Mammography Quality Standards Act requires that mammography clinics meet appropriate standards of equipment and personnel and that they be available for inspection.

The second piece of legislation supports the development of a national cancer data base. Such a base has been established by the American Cancer Society and this bill gives added financial support to their work. It also mandates investigation of geographic differences in breast cancer rates throughout our country.

––––––––––

Before a cell undergoes malignant transformation and a cancer begins, certain genetic changes take place within the cell. The cause for this change is something "new" that develops within the DNA of the cell itself and, since it is new, it therefore provides us with a "marker." The newly created cancer cell now has different DNA properties than a normal cell. This creates more new "markers," but they are after the fact—the cancer cell has already been born. Nevertheless, all these markers provide molecular biologists and geneticists with tools to detect malignant change even before it occurs!

Massive ongoing research is directed toward identifying these markers early on—CA-125 is an example of one marker-chaser. CA-125 and all the other markers we have talked about in this chapter react in the same way for all humans. Eventually there may even be a form of "cocktail" made up of several markers that can test us at one time for a number of malignant conditions.

Even more incredible research involves introducing genetically modified cells into the body that can destroy those cells in the body which are about to undergo malignant transformation. This treatment is now actually going on in a few centers throughout our country.

Reasons for having a mammogram—and for not having one—are complex and vary by race, age and economic status. Three-quarters of those women WHO HAVE mammograms say that a physician recommended the test.

Still, almost 40 percent of white American women over forty have never had a mammogram. The main given reason? Forty percent said it was not recommended by their physician. Thirty percent said it was an unnecessary test and about 5 percent balked at the cost. The figures for black American women were 52 percent, 22 percent and 2.6 percent.

The good news is that more and more women are accepting mammograms and more and more physicians are recognizing their responsibility in urging their patients on.

11

AGING—SUCCESSFULLY

"Age is something that doesn't matter—unless you are a cheese."
—Billie Burke

Would that Ms. Burke's words were right. They were spoken many years ago when there wasn't very much age to go around. Today the reality of aging with all its problems—and potential—faces an incredible and ever-increasing number of Americans.

When Julius Caesar was making his bid for world conquest, life expectancy was about twenty-eight years. At the turn of this century—over 2,000 years later—it was only forty years. But what a change this century has produced! From the introduction to our book, you already know that a female born today can plan to live well into her eighties. Maybe considerably longer—if the world is still here.

So the ranks and numbers of master citizens are mushrooming. There are over 30 million of us now and, when the baby boomers join us shortly, our cohorts will rise sharply. So sharply that in the next thirty years we will double. At least one person in seven will be over sixty-five!

In this chapter, we are going to look at some things we know and don't know about the aging process and its effects on our bodies, and how we can forcefully and actively make the major limitations of aging retreat into our distant horizons and work against our eventual rendezvous with destiny.

Some problems:

- Studies on aging in the past generally involved males confined to nursing homes and the like. The data accumulated thereby was obviusly biased and did not reflect the true aging processes. New studies are shattering many of the older, incorrect concepts that mangled and shackled our management of aging people.

- Physicians—unfortunately—have tended to address their aging practice population as a cranky, senile, demanding group of nonfunctioning citizens that they could best handle by medicating them into submission. This attitude is changing—sometimes with foot-dragging, but changing.

- Medical schools and teaching institutions have begun to grasp the importance of our large and aging population. Geriatrics is now being taught to medical students and others in the healing arts. We are also beginning to see certified "geriatricians" enter private practice throughout our country, though they are still in short supply.

- The fact that women age differently and more rapidly destructive than men is just now beginning to sink in. Thus, studies on aging as it relates to women alone are beginning. I must point out that as a specialty group, gynecologists have been way ahead of the field (and in the field I include geriatricians and internists) in initiating studies to protect women as they proceed through the senior years.

- Gender bashing and gender bias are no better demonstrated than toward aging women. In business, aging women are disproportionately discriminated against. This is a well-understood truism. Less understood is the gender bias now being demonstrated in medicine. For instance, in the current studies to cap medical care costs, serious consideration is being given to rationing and deleting medical care to our aging population. Since more of them are surviving, the vast majority of Americans thus being considered for rationed care are women.

How Aging Takes Place—the Bad News

The process by which our bodies decline is complex and involves a number of factors—some understood, some not.

- Fundamental to the aging process is a decrease in the body's ability to adapt to stress—any kind of stress—and consequently an increase in the body's vulnerability to damage. A very simple example is the body's reaction to influenza. This relatively minor infection of young people can become deadly in the older population. The body's resources to fight this infection are here marshaled more slowly and less effectively. The altered physiology behind the aging body's loss of adaptibility is not yet understood.

- Diminished faculties regularly reduce our ability to see and hear and move about. Much of this can be at least partially compensated for, but the decline continues. We become more limited in our spheres of activity and more prone to accidents and injury.

- Damage to our bodies by illness and injury as well as destructive lifelong lifestyle habits increasingly take their toll. Chronic exposure to pollutants and irritants add their chronic insults to our mainframes. Finally, we are more susceptible to chronic illnesses—arthritis, hypertension, heart disease, diabetes and more. Some of these disorders can be prevented, delayed or modified by lifestyle changes, no matter what your age.

• And in women—with its destructive consequences, the loss of protective estrogen.

Two other life factors significantly affect aging:

• *Isolation*. Maybe Lord Byron said it most sharply—but certainly most eloquently:

> "What worst of woes that wait on age?
> What stamps the wrinkle deeper on the brow?
> To view each loved one blotted from life's page
> And be alone on earth, as I am now."

That's a very forlorn, depressing passage but it speaks volumes of truth about one inescapable problem of aging.

• *Poverty*. Some aging people are well off but most are not. Social Security is the major income for over one-third of the American elderly. Clearly the social ills of poverty contribute to the speed of aging by currying immobility, malnutrition, depression and more.

All of these problems, then—and assuredly more—contribute their own weight to the progression of the aging process.

Let's proceed now to get all the bad news out of the way and then we'll move on to our success story.

The Effects of Aging on Certain Body Systems

Listed below are ways specific parts of your body and certain bodily functions react to the aging process.

The Brain

The intellectual capacities of a normal brain remain stable until we reach at least seventy. Although memory chips and cognitive chips are disappearing at the rate of 100,000 or so each day after age forty, there is a tremendous untapped reservoir of these "Golgi" (think cells) chips in brain storage, so that their loss is not deeply felt. Thus the intellectual capacities go on as always into the seventies. New research establishes quite clearly that these remaining untapped brain chips can actually be *brought on line* and utilized. That means we can rejoice in the continued *expansion* of our brainpower by simply reprogramming our software! All this, of course, can take place only in a healthy aging brain, where neurological disease has not taken an irreversible toll.

Memory—and the Loss of Memory

(This is my second go at the memory section. I forgot to save it in my word processor the first time around!) Memory is a very complex part of the human brain function and it has been poorly understood by neurological scientists. It still is, but we are learning some things:

- Loss of memory for recent events is our most common aging complaint. We can quote perfectly a sonnet memorized in the seventh grade but can't remember our stupid Medicare number or whether we flushed the toilet. This type of memory loss can be compensated for as we shall see and should not give rise to fear of organic brain disease—like Alzheimer's syndrome. Only 5 percent of memory loss problems are associated with organic brain disease.

- There are different levels of memory, different ways of transmitting memory impulses of things we both want to and don't want to remember. There are also different memory storage areas in the brain, some of which supply very transient services. And the competition may be fierce.

- Substances called neurotransmitters (NTRs) carry memory impulses to storage areas. These NTRs weaken as we age and are likely to lose impulses formerly retained. NTRs can now be made in the laboratory and their experimental use is under study.

- Medication and stress significantly interfere with memory storage.

There are ways to help minimize our memory problems and we will learn about them subsequently in the good news to follow. If I remember.

The Skeleton

As you know, bone loss begins in the thirties, accelerates rapidly during the years just after menopause, then continues at a slower pace thereafter. Fractures appear in the sixty- to eighty-year age group with nonhealing being the usual course of events. You are aware of the factors accelerating this common crippling disorder, osteoporosis.

Heart and Lungs

Much of the original data on heart and lung functioning in the later years was based on incorrect evidence obtained from sick oldsters.

While hypertension and arteriosclerosis are more likely to be present, otherwise healthy women have excellent cardiac and lung function diminished only slightly by aging—and most of that is due to inactivity. And can be reversed.

Blood

The composition of the blood is little changed as the years go by. Total blood counts of both red and white cells (except perhaps for lymphocytes) should be at the same levels as always. The bone marrow maintains its ability to replace and rebuild blood levels rapidly. Thus, anemia in a ninety-year-old woman should be thoroughly investigated since it generally signifies hidden blood loss rather than iron deficiency.

Metabolism

It is commonly accepted by doctors that as their patients age, the patients lose their ability to metabolize sugar. Thus age-onset diabetes is not an unexpected problem in the oldster. However, it now appears that sugar tolerance studies for master citizens are undoubtedly incorrect and too rigid, thus consigning innocent victims to the diabetes enclave. Moreover, the apparently age-related decline in ability to metabolize sugar often can be reversed by an increase in physical activity.

In other metabolic areas, the number of calories required to maintain body weight decreases as time goes on. Therefore, if caloric intake doesn't decline and activity levels remain the same, body weight will increase. In that regard I am not telling you anything you didn't know. But now new insurance tables come to the rescue! Guess what. The old tables were all too strict. We masters should all weigh about ten to fifteen pounds *more* than formerly advocated. Hallelujah!

Muscle Mass

As time goes by, muscle mass and strength tend to decline. This may be due to tissue aging or to the absence of male or male-like hormones. However, the weight of evidence reveals that *lack of physical activity* is the greatest thief of muscle. Thus, at almost any age, physical activity will rebuild muscle.

Sexual Organs

This has been completely covered elsewhere (page 39). Once ovarian activity ceases, women begin to have atrophy of the vulva and vagina, loss of lubrication, orgasmic delay or absence, loss of sexual fantasies and diminished sexual drive.

Skin

Your wraparound is vastly affected by any number of internal and external factors. Sunlight exposure, weight gain and loss, diet, smoking and alcohol and many other factors enter into what you have to look at each morning in the mirror. Generally, the skin ages more rapidly than other systems when it is subject to prolonged irritation. When estrogen is absent, skin collagen (supportive tissues) regularly disappears and the wrinkling rate accelerates. The greatest skin damage is probably done by sunlight; and the thinning atmosphere, combined with our sun worship, poses for us a dangerous epidemic of fatal skin cancer (melanoma). For those of you with delicate skin, remember, the porcelain look is "in." Even if sun exposure has never bothered your skin, minimize your cancer risk by staying out of the sun and tanning booths.

Teeth

Although tooth cavitation (the development of cavities) usually decreases at this time, bone erosion will often loosen teeth so that they fall out. Changes in occlusion (the way teeth fit together when the jaws are closed), caused by bone and tooth loss, also often induce gum disease and, in the past, the price was "teeth in a cup." Changing hygiene practices and modern orthodontics have reversed these unpleasant oral problems.

All our lives we have been told to brush our teeth very frequently and regularly with a good firm brush and abrasive toothpaste. By following these dental instructions, we have, over the years, brushed most of our enamel away so that even an angelhair brush with aloe-cream paste is painful to our residual nubs! But clean we must.

The Psychology of Aging

We have had a wealth of theory surrounding a poverty of solutions regarding the psychology of aging. Yet those involved in the mental health care of master citizens are beginning to recognize the following baseline psychological principles:

- Older people are generally more intelligent and worldly than those attempting to manage them. They have command, by and large, of a much greater vocabulary and have a more catholic and profound outlook on life. The fact that they may not want to take the time to share it with a neophyte does not mean it is not there. This is, of course, not always true. A fool at thirty will probably be a fool at sixty-five. (But a lot of fools are gone by sixty-five.)

- Most master citizens are proud and independent. They abhor disrespectful treatment and respond to it in kind.

Being designated by a case number, or worse still, by a first name, will draw the contempt it begs. It is worth noting that 70 percent of twenty- to twenty-five-year-olds interviewed stated that senior citizens should be cared for in their children's homes, while only 16 percent of the senior citizens agreed!

- The greatest crises that master citizens face are not challenges (career changes, for example) but losses due to death and separation as well as losses of physical function. These are the problems they most certainly and inevitably have to deal with.

Master citizens, then, wish to preserve their identity and have the liberty to be their "eccentric" selves, but need compassionate, nonpatronizing help in managing the gradual loss of all things they hold dear.

Lifestyles for the Long Haul— the Good News

At long last the misery is behind us and we can look forward to a pleasurable winter harvest. To begin with, nowhere is the old maxim "Use it or lose it" more applicable. We have seen that many of our parts that were supposed to wither and crumble away can indeed be maintained—even restarted—by a proper LIFESTYLE and a POSITIVE approach. Thus, pushing, prodding and pumping our brains, our muscles and our cardiovascular systems will not only maintain our status quo but will cause our bodies to respond continuously with further growth.

Here is *THE PLAN:*

Our Daily Bread

What to eat and drink has been hammered home all through your book so no big dissertation is needed here—only some gentle reminders.

- A balanced low-fat (20 percent only, and nonsaturated) diet is the key. Follow our new outline, which raises animal fat and dairy products almost to the treat level. Balanced means adequate fresh produce, beans, lentils, peas and cereal groups along with complex carbohydrates. Bulk is increasingly important and may require the addition of bulking agents (Metamucil, etc.).

- Keep your calories at a level that maintains your best weight—and no more.

- The colon may resist digesting some highly seasoned and rich foods so adored in the good old days. Abdominal bloating and pain should warn you away.

- Whiskey in moderation has many therapeutic effects. Red wine in moderation is apparently cardioprotective. Remember: Alcohol is no problem when it's no problem.

Exercise

Here, again, there is little to add—only to reinforce.

- If you have had a lifestyle of programmed exercise you know your limits and what you need to do to continue to thrive.

- A mix of aerobic exercises, walking and bicycling are important. Also, to maintain muscle strength some resistance training is important.

- An exercise program is best when it is constructive, interesting and rewarding. Many other programs fall by the wayside. Thus, bricklaying (you can do it!), real gardening and many competitive sports provide exercise, companionship and fulfillment. Better than riding a stationary bike!

Habits

- There is no need to say don't smoke and don't do illegal drugs. You won't. And if you do, please get some help to quit. There are many resources available.

- If you are not an alcoholic and have no restrictive medical problems, you can enjoy the multiple benefits of moderate alcohol without any fear and with pleasure.

Sex

- Nowhere is "use it or lose it" more germane. If you have an acceptable, secure sexual outlet, do everything you can to keep it going. HRT and local estrogen help to preserve what's involved. Masturbation by whatever method is not immoral, but avoid kinky equipment that can hurt.

Hygiene

- Involuntary spillage from the bladder and the intestines make frequent fastidious showering important for a sense of cleanliness as well as the prevention of perineal skin damage and irritation that can become a severe constant nuisance.

- Because of the as yet unexplained risk of ovarian cancer, don't use talcum powder around the vagina.

• Painful teeth or not, use a water-pressure cleaning device regularly and softly brush your teeth several times daily.

Medications and your Physician

Avoid as many medications as you can. Many times the following suggestions will eliminate the need for some medicines:

• Throw out old drugs. Don't try anyone else's and be sure you understand the need for your own. Also be aware of your medication's side effects and any potential interaction with other drugs.

• If you have several physicians in various specialties, be sure that each one is aware of *all* the medications that you are taking.

• Take medication exactly as directed. More is not better. Don't restart any on your own.

• Independent studies show that your gynecologist treats you more holistically than any other physician. So bond with her and see her regularly. Tell her what is really going on—lay it *all* out. Get your mammogram and Pap smear regularly along with whatever other screening tests she advises. Continue with HRT indefinitely unless you are provided with a valid reason to stop it. "I think it's time to quit" is not a valid reason.

Traveling

When you go to the sun spots, the snow spots or the night spots of the world, there are some bad spots to consider.

• Protect yourself against sunlight. The risk of skin cancer has become too great.

- Going from near sea level to a high environment, pace yourself slowly for the first few days.

- Don't drive at night or for long periods of time.

- If you have to fly more than two continuous hours get up and move around as vigorously as you can. Keep the circulation in your legs going.

- When traveling outside the country remember that the food may be older than the wine. Master citizens are sensitive to foreign bacteria in their food and water. Be careful and carry Bactrim with you for traveler's diarrhea unless you are allergic to sulfa medication.

- Although most of us are not disabled, the Americans with Disabilities Act has made it easier for us to get in and around Taj Mahal–like hotels that glory in deep high-entry steps, raucous dark foyers and restaurants, chairs that scrape bottom and dimly lit interiors. Most bathrooms are poorly illuminated on the belief that we are ashamed or afraid to see ourselves in them! Enforced change is coming.

Thinking and Remembering

- Work your brain. Either alone or in the company of others plan, write, think, investigate, solve problems and puzzles, read and communicate. Don't vegetate—activate and circulate.

- Watch medications—many of them affect memory. Ask.

- Avoid distractions when you are memorizing—or trying to.

- *Listen* and *focus*.

- Maintain lists. Leave things in the same place.

- Don't try to memorize junk—it competes for space.

- Keep your brain involved as suggested above. That helps keep circuits going and opens new ones that have never been used. There is still room for rent! And it is user-friendly.

If you are worried about memory loss, don't. Even though worry is a good sign! Those of us losing memory because of severe organic brain disease truly don't worry about it. The ability to worry has been destroyed.

Work

Yes—work. Think about it. An idle mind is the devil's workshop and an idle body is his pantry. Old and trite—but true. Doctor Howard Shapiro defines our work best: ". . . one way to feel young is to have projects and goals. The old add contemplation to the stimulation of work. We are, after all, in no hurry" (*Drug Therapy*, November 1990).

Coping

Isolation, separation, fear and depression—these are all real things that haunt us more as time goes by. Since they are real, they need to be dealt with as intensely as all our other challenges. Many of the goals and plans that we have already investigated and listed will provide us with strong support here. But there is more:

- Networking is a basic tool. Through work, clubs, church, AARP, family and friendships comes a supporting network that is an important bridgehead to ultimate peace and security.

• Faith. Networking is a human and imperfect bridgehead. It is, after all, made up of us. Faith carries us over the bridge into peace—peace that passes our understanding.

• Power. It is all around us. Faith allows us to draw upon it and leads us beyond the bridgehead.

We have talked about these things before—but nothing is more important. And there is no other way.

Vaya con Dios.

ℰ Pause and Reflect

As you are now aware, aging affects our reaction to stress of all kinds—and vice versa. One of the greatest of all stresses that we face at any age is emotional stress caused by life situations.

If we say the death of a spouse is rated as 100 on our stress scale, then what values, relative to that, do other stressful situations have?

> Divorce: 70
> Death of a close family member: 63
> Jail: 63
> Major personal injury or illness: 53
> Getting fired: 47
> Retirement: 45
> Sexual problems: 39
> Death of a close friend: 37
> In-law troubles: 29

The list goes on.

———————

The incidence of depression is increasing worldwide. No one knows why, but it is a fact. Here are some interesting things you may want to know about depression:

- A major episode of depression in a woman born in the 1930s will most likely occur as she nears fifty. However, if depression occurs in a woman born in the 1950s, it will most likely happen when she is about thirty.

- Although experts have long pooh-poohed the notion that estrogen and testosterone have any value in the management of depression, it has recently been established that such is the case. These steroid sex hormones play a distinct role in the control of related depressive problems.

- An interesting study, initiated by the National Institute of Mental Health, provided three separate categories of treatment at various institutions for depressed patients. The first two groups were exposed to two different types of psychotherapy, the third to antidepressant drug therapy or an inert placebo. The results? The drug therapy worked more rapidly and more effectively than psychotherapy. The placebo failed, but not completely. While the three groups each eventually had about a 60 percent cure rate, the placebo helped almost 30 percent of those who took it.

Outward Bound is an organization that dumps acceptable volunteer groups or individuals—for a price—into the wilderness with a minimum of equipment and a maximum of advice. The game is to get back to civilization intact and self-confident. Master citizens, who are mainly self-confident to begin with, are accepted for this program when they qualify. Many older people participate simply to prove their independence and enjoy doing it.

———————

A popular misconception is that earlier generations were far more devoted to their elders than children are today. This stereotype is just not true. For instance:

- About 78 percent of all adults over eighty-five live in their own homes or with relatives.

- An estimated five million Americans provide parental care in some way on any given day.

- Over 70 percent of the 2.2 million Americans who provide care to the frail elderly are women (23 percent are wives, 29 percent daughters, 19 percent other females). Their average age is fifty-seven, but fully one-third of them are over sixty-five. Of the daughters who provide care, 44 percent work outside of their homes, while 11 percent quit work to provide full-time care. Nearly one-third are poor—or near poor.

The enormous sacrifices that these caregivers are making has only recently been recognized. Their efforts to make living as normal as possible for aging relatives deserves our recognition and respect.

———————

The United Nations Vienna International Plan of Action on Aging in 1982 proposed ten basic principles to be observed for the care of the elderly, namely:

Equality, individuality, independence, choice, mobility, productivity, home-care, access to services, cohesion among generations and promotion of self-care and family care.

Even the narrowest achievement of these goals will require a great deal of energy and money, which is often channeled elsewhere. For instance, developed nations spent about $345 billion on military matters in 1978 and, during the same year, about $213 billion on health goals. Developing countries, on the other hand, spent $102 billion on arms and only $22 billion on health care matters!

It is worth noting that the United States contributed .23%—less than one-quarter of one percent—of the gross national product for the development of the aging care goals to the United Nations Organization for Economic Cooperation and Development. That represents the *lowest* contribution of *any developed nation.* The highest (1.02 percent) was from the Netherlands, followed by Norway (.99 percent) and Denmark (.85 percent). Saudia Arabia and Kuwait, the two grand champions of OPEC, contributed 3.5 percent and 4.5 percent, respectively, of their gross national products to provide the same assistance to other developing countries in their sphere of influence.

———————

Your chances of living to be one hundred are about 1 in 1,000 if you live in the United States. More women live to be centenarians than do men and their chances are greatest in Hawaii (1,713 in 100,000), Minnesota (1,444), South Dakota (1,392), Iowa (1,379), Nebraska (1,364), North Dakota (1,362), Kansas (1,339), Florida (1,336), Idaho (1,329) and Arizona (1,317).

———————

In two separate and controlled studies, intercessory prayers were shown to improve significantly patient outcome and decrease recovery time. The prayers were offered without the recipient's knowledge or request.

———————

Let's end our book lightly.

There are humorous implications in people's names. Here's some about doctor's names.

- There are eighteen doctors in this country named Doctor. So we have Doctor Doctor. Moreover, there are at least three named Doctor Nurse.

- There are twenty-two doctors variously named Needle, Probe, Lance and Ligate.

- There are nineteen named Fix, Cure and Heal.

- Nine are named either Klutz, Croak, Blunt or Blewitt.

- An orthopedist is named Bone, a rheumatologist named Knee, an anesthesiologist named Gass, a psychiatrist named Couch and a dermatologist named—you guessed it—Rash!

- There are no doctors named Placebo!

(From the *Journal of the American Medical Association,* December 1992)

QUESTIONS AND ANSWERS

Where does the word "menopause" come from?

In 1812 the French gynecologist C.P.L. Gardanne wrote a monograph dealing in its entirety with the change of life. In it he coined the word "ménépausie," which he derived from two Greek words meaning "month" and "terminate."

When does the menopause start?

Usually the menopause starts in the late forties, but there are wide variations that are within normal limits.

Can I predict when the menopause will start?

The onset of menopause can be predicted only when your ovaries must be removed for some serious disorder. The menopause will begin the next day no matter what your age. Otherwise there is no way to know when it will begin.

206

What sets it off?

The decline of ovarian hormone secretion.

How will I know when I have entered the menopause?

By the onset of a group of symptoms usually including hot flashes (flushes), night sweats, insomnia, depression, fatigue and other seemingly unrelated symptoms. Sooner or later there will also be changes in your menstrual function, changes that can be variable.

How will my doctor know I have entered the menopause?

By listening to your account of your symptoms and by certain blood tests.

What is the perimenopause?

It is a descriptive term for the few years immediately preceding the menopause. During this time, the premenstrual syndrome (PMS) may be accentuated and prolonged and certain metabolic changes, such as stepped-up calcium loss, may also begin.

When does the perimenopause start?

Usually two to three years before the menopause.

When does it end?

It folds into the menopause.

Is there a distinct line between the menopause and the perimenopause?

None at all. They are a continuum.

Why does premature menopause occur?

Any condition that prematurely stops the ovaries from making estrogen will induce a premature menopause. So the premature destruction of the ovaries by disease or infection or the premature surgical removal of the ovaries for whatever reason will induce an early menopause. Certain inherited disorders as well as some severe systemic illnesses will also accomplish the same thing.

How do I know if premature menopause is happening to me?

You will have the typical signs and symptoms of the menopause.

What is the difference between temporary ovarian failure and permanent ovarian failure?

Temporary failure can occur under periods of stress and illness. By definition, recovery will occur when the offending condition is corrected. Permanent ovarian failure is, as the name suggests, an irreversible cessation of ovarian function for whatever reason.

Will the menopause be as uncomfortable as I hear it will be?

That depends on what you hear and the circumstances of your own menopause. Generally speaking, though, almost all disturbing menopausal problems can be safely and effectively controlled with adequate hormone replacement.

How does PMS relate to the menopause?

Generally PMS symptoms, if present at all, become somewhat accentuated and prolonged as the menopause draws near.

How does a hysterectomy affect the menopause?

A hysterectomy (an operation that removes the uterus only) stops all menstrual flow permanently and produces permanent sterility. It has no direct effect on the menopause except that all problems related to the bleeding certainly cease.

How will the menopause affect my sex life?

Most commonly there is a gradual decline in sex drive, sex fantasy and vaginal lubrication along with an increase in time-to-orgasm. In later, postmenopausal years the vagina becomes very thin and dry, making sexual intercourse painful. All this assumes there has been no hormone replacement.

Do I need to continue using birth control during the menopause?

You need to practice birth control until you have not menstruated for one year. Special circumstances (hormone replacement, for instance) may alter that rule. Your doctor will know.

What role do oral contraceptives play in the menopause?

Under the proper conditions, birth control pills may be used at the menopause not only as a contraceptive but also as a menopausal hormone supplement. Mainly, to use birth control pills you must not smoke, should not have significant hypertension and must have a satisfactory experience with both their menopausal and birth control effects.

Will I gain weight during the menopause?

You can, but it will most likely be due to other body changes that occur in the middle years. Men have middle-age spread, too, but don't have a menopause. Almost anything that happens during the menopause is blamed on the menopause.

How often should I see my doctor during the menopause?

If there are no specific medical problems related to the menopause or some other gynecological condition, once a year is adequate. Otherwise, your doctor will advise you.

Do you recommend any annual tests?

A Pap smear should be performed each year, whether the cervix is in or not. Some say this is not necessary but you are asking me, not them. If there is no family history of breast cancer, a mammogram should be obtained every two years in the forties and every year thereafter. Again, you are asking me. Blood lipid tests, colon and ovarian cancer screening, bone-density studies and other tests are performed at varying time intervals, depending on many circumstances.

How important is hormone replacement therapy?

It is less important than insulin for a diabetic, but it is as important as any replacement therapy that you might ever be involved with.

Isn't hormone replacement therapy filled with risks?

No, it is not. In ordinary circumstances, the benefits vastly outweigh the few risks involved.

How is hormone replacement administered?

It may be given orally as tablets, by injection under the skin either by shots or pellets or across the skin (transdermally), using abdominal patches or vaginal creams.

How far into the menopause should I start hormone replacement therapy?

As soon as you have symptoms.

Will hormone therapy help to stabilize my mood swings?

Yes.

How much does hormone replacement therapy cost?

Depending on what method you use and whether or not you substitute generic products, from $10.00 to $20.00 per month.

Should I continue hormone replacement after the menopause?

Yes. For how long, however, depends upon many factors only you and your doctor can resolve.

Should I take vitamins during the menopause?

You are probably asking about combination vitamin and mineral preparations. Most diets adequately provide most vitamins and minerals, but you need to be sure that you have a little extra iron until menstruation ceases and that you take a calcium supplement always. An ordinary once-a-day vitamin supplement is very adequate and, after menstruation ceases, just a once-a-day vitamin pill plus a calcium supplement.

What is the postmenopause?

These are the years that follow the more or less acute time of the menopause, when menses are about to end and when the many other symptoms related to the menopause (flushing and so on) have largely abated or disappeared.

When does the postmenopause start?

As noted above, when the acute menopause phase subsides.

When does it end?

It doesn't end—rather, it continues.

Is there a distinct line between the menopause and postmenopause?

No. The one flows slowly into the other as the perimenopause flows into the menopause.

What role does estrogen play in the postmenopausal years?

In most instances it has an important role in maintaining bone strength, delaying hardening of the arteries and supporting vaginal health as well as sexual drive.

What role does progesterone play in the postmenopause?

It continues to protect the uterus and, perhaps, the breasts against the unopposed irritation that estrogen by itself has upon these organs. Further, it may help build new bone.

How are estrogen and progesterone interrelated?

They are both secreted from maturing egg follicles in the ovary and are very closely related steroid hormones.

How will a lack of estrogen affect me physically and emotionally?

Without estrogen, menses cease and the vagina atrophies. Equally, the breasts atrophy as does the skin. The rate of bone loss accelerates and the rate of arterial hardening increases. Emotionally, depression increases and sex drive decreases. Hot flushes and emotional instability along with fatigue and many other general systemic complaints become the rule.

How does testosterone figure into the hormone replacement program?

Testosterone (the male hormone) is a sexual stimulant for both men and women. Healthy ovaries secrete testosterone-like hormones, which act as a sexual stimulant. After the menopause, these hormones are often not present, and so testosterone is added to certain hormone replacement programs to supply this need.

How does nutrition affect the whole menopausal-postmenopausal complex?

Proper nutrition is always important. During these times in a woman's life, however, an adequate diet is even more important. Your food must supply most basic needs and your supplements, the rest. Animal fats and salt must be restricted to help avoid hypertension and other vascular disease and, finally, the number of calories must be decreased as body needs decrease so that obesity does not follow.

How is exercise important in the whole menopausal-postmenopausal complex?

Proper exercise plays many roles at this time. It helps in maintaining bone strength, it burns off excess calories and it vastly improves cardio-pulmonary strength and reserves. It also promotes a sense of well-being at any time.

How can I tell if I am at risk for osteoporosis?

Factors that promote the onset of osteoporosis include a family history of the condition, a very early menopause, a thin body, a fair complexion, an inactive lifestyle, an alcohol or tobacco habit and an inadequate diet. There are a few others, but these are the main risk factors.

How can I prevent osteoporosis?

By an adequate diet, including proper calcium supplements, by an active ongoing exercise program and by supplementation with HRT. Avoidance of all tobacco and of excess alcohol is also very important.

What role does calcium play in osteoporosis?

Adequate calcium intake is necessary to keep up with calcium loss. Bones lose calcium very rapidly in the early years of the menopause and postmenopause. It must be replaced. However, calcium supplementation is useless at this time without accompanying estrogen.

What are my chances of developing a breast disorder?

You have about a fifty-fifty chance of developing some minor breast disorder. Fortunately, however, breast cancer—the most serious breast disorder—will occur in just about 10 percent of all women today. That is still much too high a figure, but great hope of abatement is on the horizon.

How important are mammograms?

Just about as important as breathing. At this moment, only mammograms done as and when directed by the American Cancer Society can arrest this most disabling female cancer. Regular mammograms and Pap smears are so important to you that it is hard to equate them in importance with anything else you may do.

OUTTAKES

Perimenopause (PeriMPX)

Definition: A period of time immediately preceeding the true menopause, when certain menopausal characteristics may appear.

Cause: The beginning decline of ovarian function.

Time frame: Usually two or three years' duration.

Symptoms: An increase in the intensity and/or duration of premenstrual syndrome (PMS), fatigue, rarely premenstrual flushing, sometimes declining sexual interest.

Progression: PeriMPX symptoms generally increase as menopause approaches.

Diagnosis: Usually by patient's symptoms. Sometimes cessation of ovulation can be determined by certain tests.

Treatment: Medical management of PMS symptoms, hormone replacement therapy (HRT) if necessary, lifestyle changes, including diet and exercise and counseling.

Outcome: Good response to adequate therapy and advancement into the menopause.

Menopause (MPX)

Definition: The time of cessation of menstruation and the emotional and physical changes that accompany it.

Cause: The cessation of ovarian function and, thus, of hormone production.

Time frame: Usually between age forty-five and fifty-five and lasting several years.

Symptoms: Irregularity in, and finally absence of, menstrual bleeding, along with flushes, sweats, insomnia, depression, irritability, headaches, palpitations and numerous other less-common symptoms.

Diagnosis: Through patient's history, laboratory tests for declining estrogen production, absence of ovulation and elevated pituitary levels of follicle stimulating hormone (FSH).

Treatment: Hormone replacement therapy when physician and patient agree and when therapy is not contraindicated, plus counseling in diet, exercise and many other aspects of mature living.

Outcome: Gradual and peaceful progression into the post-menopausal years.

Postmenopause (PMPX)

Definition: All of the years following the acute menopausal events.

Cause: Virtually complete absence of the ovarian hormones, estrogen and progesterone.

Time frame: As indicated above—all the years following the menopause.

Symptoms and signs: Increasingly rapid arteriosclerosis (hardening of the arteries), osteoporosis with all its bony frame damage, declining sexual drive and thinning of the vaginal lining, which results in lubrication failure and, often, painful lovemaking.

Diagnosis: Through continuing high blood FSH levels along with low estrogen levels, low vaginal estrogen smears, evidence of increasing arteriosclerosis and osteoporosis, patient's symptoms.

Management: HRT, calcium supplementation, diet, exercise and adequate counseling.

Outcome: A gentle and safe journey into maturity.

GLOSSARY

Words in SMALL CAPITAL LETTERS are also entries in this glossary.

adrenal glands: ENDOCRINE glands that secrete hormones into the body. The adrenal hormones are mainly adrenalin and COR-TISONE, but the glands are also capable of making a TESTOSTER-ONE-like hormone. There is an adrenal gland sitting on top of each kidney.

amenorrhea: The absence of MENSTRUATION.

androstenedione: A hormone substance made in the ADRENAL GLANDS and in the OVARIES. It resembles the male hormone TES-TOSTERONE in many of its actions.

anemia: A decrease in the red blood cell count below acceptable limits. Anemia may be due to blood loss, an iron-deficient diet or a number of systemic disorders.

arteriosclerosis: The deposition of calcium plaques along the ar-terial walls, also known as hardening of the arteries. This aging process is accelerated by high cholesterol blood levels and by smoking.

breast self-examination: The technique of examining one's own breasts. The technique, which should be done monthly, may be learned from a physician, from mammogram clinics, hospital wellness centers and pamphlets put out by the American Cancer Society and other agencies.

calcium: A mineral element fundamental for normal body function. The daily diet should include 1000 mg of calcium in order to satisfy bone, muscle and blood needs.

calcitonin: A hormone secreted by the parafollicular cells of the THYROID GLAND, another ENDOCRINE organ. Calcitonin is important in regulating the storage of CALCIUM in bone.

climacteric: Another term for the MENOPAUSE. The term is not very popular, so it is not used very often.

corpus luteum: A mass of hormone-secreting tissue in the ovary. After OVULATION occurs, the granulosal cells that surrounded the maturing egg and made ESTROGEN are converted to lutein cells and begin to secrete PROGESTERONE. These remnant cells remain organized in a cyst-like cavity called the corpus luteum ("yellow body"). The whole structure disintegrates just before MENSTRUATION.

cortical bone: Thick, smooth, hard plates of dense bone, as opposed to honey-combed TRABECULAR bone. The outside long shafts of the bones in our extremities are perfect examples of cortical bone.

cortisone: A very powerful hormone secreted from the ADRENAL GLANDS and needed for the proper function of many body systems. It is often used in medicine to treat serious disorders of body function, certain autoimmune diseases, some arthritis and serious allergic disorders.

endocrine glands: Glands that secrete hormones internally. The hormones then go somewhere else to do their work. Included here are the ADRENALS, OVARIES and testicles, THYROID, PARATHYROID, PITUITARY and certain others.

endometriosis: A disorder of the pelvic organs where little blood cysts made up of ENDOMETRIUM cells are found on the uterus, tubes, ovaries, pelvic ligaments and even bladder and bowel wall. It is a painful condition because these little blood cysts menstruate internally each month and grow a little bigger. It is associated with infertility.

endometrium: The normal lining of the uterine cavity that grows each month under the influence of ESTROGEN and PROGESTERONE and then partially menstruates away unless pregnancy has occurred.

estradiol (E2): One of the two main ESTROGENS. Almost all E2 is made within the ovary.

estrogen: The basic female hormone produced by the OVARIES in a monthly pattern throughout the reproductive years. An integral part of HRT (HORMONE REPLACEMENT THERAPY).

estrone (E1): One of the two main ESTROGENS. It is largely made from ESTRADIOL (E2).

flushes: In the MENOPAUSE, a feeling of heat and warmth, beginning somewhere deep inside and resulting in a flushed and red face. An individual flush lasts several minutes.

follicle stimulating hormone (FSH): One of several PITUITARY hormones that stimulates the OVARIES. Each month FSH initiates maturation of a capable follicle so that it prepares for OVULA-

TION. FSH also stimulates the granulosal cells in each maturing follicle to make ESTROGEN.

hormone replacement therapy (HRT): When the ovaries cease to function adequately, or if they have been removed surgically, HRT with proper amounts of ESTROGEN and PROGESTERONE is given to fill the void created.

hormone smear: A test used to determine estrogen levels in the body. Estrogen stimulates the vaginal lining to grow, and it maintains the lining in a mature, healthy state. Smears taken from the vaginal wall and stained reveal the degree of maturity, and a count of these scraped-off cells is called a maturation index. This index is a general indicator of estrogen levels in the body.

hysterectomy: The removal of the uterus, whether done abdominally or vaginally.

luteinizing hormone (LH): A powerful PITUITARY hormone that surges out somewhere around the middle of a regular menstrual cycle. It forces the mature follicle to OVULATE and stimulates development of the CORPUS LUTEUM. Modern home ovulation-predictor kits can identify this LH surge and thus predict ovulation a few hours before it happens.

mammography: An x-ray technique that, using very minimal radiation, detects serious breast disease at a much earlier time and with much greater accuracy than any other single or combined examination or test.

mastectomy: The surgical removal of a breast. A radical mastectomy is the removal of a breast along with associated and surrounding muscle, gland tissues and skin.

menarche: The beginning of MENSTRUATION.

menopause (MPX): The mid-life cessation of MENSES and the attendant body changes associated with it and around it.

menses: See MENSTRUATION.

menstruation: The regular monthly flow of blood and tissue debris from the uterus.

MPX: A common abbreviation signifying MENOPAUSE.

myomata: Fibrous muscular tumors that quite commonly grow upon and within the uterine walls. Almost always benign, these tumors may get very large and may cause heavy, painful uterine bleeding. Also commonly called *fibroids*.

night sweats: Hot flashes that occur during the night. Usually the intense heat makes you push your covers back and you awaken cooled by the sweat evaporating on your now-exposed skin.

osteoporosis: A condition characterized by the decrease in bone mass that results in frailty of the bones. When CALCIUM leaves bone, for whatever reason, the bone becomes weakened and osteoporosis exists. There are many causes of osteoporosis, simple aging being one of them. The loss of ESTROGEN at the MENOPAUSE, however, is by far the commonest and most serious cause of osteoporosis. Without estrogen, calcium leaves the bone at a very rapid rate.

ovary: The female sex gland. The ovaries are responsible for more or less regular OVULATION and for the secretion of ESTROGEN, PROGESTERONE and certain other hormones into the circulation.

ovulation: The releasing of an egg from the OVARY into the peritoneal cavity, which surrounds or encloses all abdominal organs.

oxytocin: A PITUITARY hormone that affects the reproductive organs. Oxytocin makes the uterine muscle contract vigorously.

Thus it is important during labor. This hormone also helps initiate lactation.

Pap smear: A smear taken from the uterine cervix, stained and examined in a way perfected by a Greek-born American anatomist, George Papanicolaou. This smear, taken on a regular basis, has saved millions of women from cancer of the cervix. At present there is a virtual epidemic of cancer of the cervix in our youngsters. This is due to the widespread presence of the human papilloma virus (HPV) in the teenage population. It is a sexually transmitted virus that lives in the vagina and cervix and in the male's sexual anatomy. It is very important, then, that all sexually active youngsters have regular (at least annual) Pap smears.

parathyroid glands: A series of tiny ENDOCRINE GLANDS lying behind the THYROID. They secrete substances that control CALCIUM metabolism and balance.

perimenopause (PeriMPX): The two- to three-year period before the menopause, when some signs of declining hormone production begin to appear. The PREMENSTRUAL SYNDROME, for instance, should it be present, tends to intensify. These years, for descriptive and clinical purposes, have been designated the PeriMPX.

pituitary gland: The master ENDOCRINE GLAND. Its secretions control and affect all the other glands and many basic body functions. Much of this gland's power remains a mystery.

postmenopause (PMPX): After the more or less acute years of MENSES cessation and after the visceral symptoms (FLUSHES, for example) subside, the postmenopause begins. And it comprises all the years that follow.

premature menopause: The cessation of MENSES before forty accompanied by typical menopausal symptoms. There are many causes.

premature ovarian failure: As the name suggests, the failure of the ovaries to function prior to the established time of MENO-PAUSE. This may be temporary and due to stress of various sorts or severe illnesses—but recovery is the rule. Or it may be permanent and become a premature menopause. There are several causes.

premenstrual syndrome (PMS): A very complex set of disorders that precedes MENSTRUATION by a variable number of days. Depression, irritability, swelling, breast tenderness, headaches and many other symptoms characterize this common condition. The treatment is varied and not uniformly successful.

primary osteoporosis: Bone loss that occurs with aging or with ESTROGEN deficiency.

progestagens: Synthetic hormones that resemble PROGESTERONE closely, both in their chemical makeup and in their effects upon the female body. Also called progestins.

progesterone: An important female hormone produced in the OVARIES. It is secreted by lutein cells found in the CORPUS LU-TEUM cyst, which is a normal structure formed at the site of OVU-LATION and which has a lifespan of about two weeks. It is important for normal MENSTRUATION, for the maintenance of pregnancy (if one should occur, the corpus luteum lives on) and to combat the irritative action of ESTROGEN on the ENDOME-TRIUM and other tissues.

progestin: See PROGESTAGENS.

prolactin: A hormone made by the PITUITARY gland. Normally, it supports lactation, but when overproduced by certain pituitary abnormalities, it can arrest all menstrual function.

secondary osteoporosis: The form of bone weakening and demineralization that is always secondary to some other disorder.

Many glandular and bone diseases can produce this form of bone weakness.

steroids: Variations of a chemical configuration made by the body from cholesterol that result in all the sex hormones and most adrenal hormones.

temporary ovarian failure: The shutting down or diminishing of ovarian function for a period of time. Stress—such as that caused by excessive exercise, bulemia or anorexia and life situations of many kinds—can halt ovarian activity for a period of time. Moreover, many severe illnesses can do the same thing. As the term implies, ovarian recovery will follow removal of the cause.

testosterone: The male hormone secreted by the testicles and, perhaps, in small amounts, by certain other tissues in both men and women.

thenarche: The beginning of breast buds and breast development. This usually precedes the menarche (beginning of MENSTRUATION) by a few years.

thyroid gland: As part of the ENDOCRINE system, the thyroid gland secretes thyroid hormone into the bloodstream, and this hormone regulates all body metabolism. The thyroid gland also secretes CALCITONIN, which helps control CALCIUM activity in the body.

trabecular bone: The honey-combed bone girders found inside the firm shafts of exterior CORTICAL BONE. Look in the center of the bone in a T-bone steak and you will see trabecular bone.

INDEX

About the Author

Dr. Gillespie was born in North Bay, Ontario, Canada, and educated at McGill University in Montreal. His training in obstetrics and gynecology was completed in the United States and he now lives and practices in Little Rock, Arkansas. Dr. Gillespie is certified by the American Board of Obstetrics and Gynecology and is a Fellow of the American College of Obstetricians and Gynecologists. In 1977 he was elected a Fellow of the Royal College of Obstetricians and Gynecologists in London, England, an unusual honor for American citizens. Besides maintaining his private practice he serves as clinical professor of obstetrics and gynecology at the University of Arkansas School of Medicine. He is a member of a number of scientific societies and has received awards for his research from the American Medical Association, the Southern Medical Association, the American Fertility Society and the Pacific Coast Fertility Society.

Dr. Gillespie is the author of numerous scientific publications, as well as *Your Pregnancy Month by Month* and *Primelife Pregnancy*.